Thieme

# Spine Essentials Handbook

## A Bulleted Review of Anatomy, Evaluation, Imaging, Tests, and Procedures

**Kern Singh, MD**
Professor
Department of Orthopaedic Surgery
Co-Director, Minimally Invasive Spine Institute
Rush University Medical Center
Chicago, Illinois

**165 illustrations**

Thieme
New York • Stuttgart • Delhi • Rio de Janeiro

Executive Editor: William Lamsback
Managing Editor: Nikole Y. Connors
Director, Editorial Services: Mary Jo Casey
Production Editor: Naamah Schwartz
International Production Director: Andreas Schabert
Editorial Director: Sue Hodgson
International Marketing Director: Fiona Henderson
International Sales Director: Louisa Turrell
Director of Institutional Sales: Adam Bernacki
Senior Vice President and Chief Operating Officer: Sarah
   Vanderbilt
President: Brian D. Scanlan

Illustrations drawn by Andrea Hines and Alyssa Minatel

**Library of Congress Cataloging-in-Publication Data**

Names: Singh, Kern, editor.
Title: Spine essentials handbook : a bulleted reviewof
   anatomy, evaluation, imaging, tests, and procedures /
   Kern Singh, MD.
Description: First edition. | New York : Thieme, [2019] |
   Includes bibliographical references. |
Identifiers: LCCN 2018041349 (print) | LCCN
   2018047944 (ebook) | ISBN 9781626235106 (e-book) |
   ISBN 9781626235076 (print) | ISBN 9781626235106
   (ebook)
Subjects: LCSH: Spine—Surgery—Handbooks, manuals, etc.
Classification: LCC RD768 (ebook) | LCC RD768 .S6744
   2019 (print) | DDC 617.5/6059—dc23
LC record available at https://lccn.loc.gov/2018041349

© 2019 Thieme Medical Publishers, Inc.

Thieme Publishers New York
333 Seventh Avenue, New York, NY 10001 USA
+1 800 782 3488, customerservice@thieme.com

Thieme Publishers Stuttgart
Rüdigerstrasse 14, 70469 Stuttgart, Germany
+49 [0]711 8931 421, customerservice@thieme.de

Thieme Publishers Delhi
A-12, Second Floor, Sector-2, Noida-201301
Uttar Pradesh, India
+91 120 45 566 00, customerservice@thieme.in

Thieme Publishers Rio de Janeiro, Thieme Publicações
   Ltda.
Edifício Rodolpho de Paoli, 25º andar
Av. Nilo Peçanha, 50 – Sala 2508,
Rio de Janeiro 20020-906 Brasil
+55 21 3172-2297 / +55 21 3172-1896
www.thiemerevinter.com.br

Cover design: Thieme Publishing Group
Typesetting by DiTech Process Solutions

Printed in Germany by Beltz Grafische Betriebe    5 4 3

ISBN 978-1-62623-507-6

Also available as an e-book:
eISBN 978-1-62623-510-6

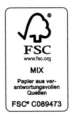

I dedicate this book to my father. As I now progress into parenthood, I realize the sacrifices you made for me. Never ending patience, bountiful amounts of time, and a dedication to giving me every opportunity to succeed.

*- K. Singh*

# Associate Editors

**Brittany E. Haws, MD**
Orthopedic Surgery Resident
University of Rochester
Rochester, New York

**Fady Y. Hijji, MD**
Orthopedic Surgery Resident
Wright State University
Dayton, Ohio

**Benjamin Khechen, BA**
Research Coordinator
Rush University Medical Center
Chicago, Illinois

**Ankur S. Narain, MD**
Orthopedic Surgery Resident
University of Massachusetts
Boston, Massachusetts

**Dil V. Patel, BS**
Research Coordinator
Rush University Medical Center
Chicago, Illinois

# Contents

# Preface

The *Spine Essentials Handbook* was produced as a portable resource that is easily accessible to all medical professionals. The detailed information, ranging from basic neuroanatomy to spinal pathology to surgical intervention, allows the reader to fully grasp the complexity of the spine. This holistic compilation helps the audience become comfortable with the intricacy of the spine before entering a clinic or the operating room. The clear depiction of complex spinal anatomy overlaid with real-time intraoperative pictures facilitates an understanding of the nuances associated with spine surgery. As any surgery demands efficiency, the accompanying text provides an in-depth coverage of technique as well as pearls to help execute the operation expeditiously. Lastly, the handbook outlines possible complications associated with spine surgery with suggestions for prevention.

The text offers up-to-date knowledge in the quickly advancing field of spinal anatomy, pathology, and surgery. With comprehensive images, cross-sectional illustrations, and emphasis on potential difficulties, this handbook allows for improved expertise on surgical procedures and postoperative care. Clinical questions included in the electronic version of the book are provided to help test and solidify your knowledge and comprehension about the complexities of spine and spinal surgery.

This handbook will be of value to not only surgeons and surgical trainees, but also for the other surgical staff involved in the medical care of spine surgery patients. We are optimistic that the *Spine Essentials Handbook* will grant readers a better understanding of the delicacies of spine surgery.

*Kern Singh, MD*

# Acknowledgements

We would like to thank all of those who assisted in the creation of this book. In particular, we would like to acknowledge Brittany Haws and Benjamin Khechen for their efforts in seeing this book to completion.

# Contributors

Ikechukwu Achebe, BS
Department of Orthopaedic Surgery
Rush University Medical Center
Chicago, Illinois

Junyoung Ahn, MD
Department of Orthopaedic Surgery
Rush University Medical Center
Chicago, Illinois

Daniel D. Bohl, MS, MD
Department of Orthopaedic Surgery
Rush University Medical Center
Chicago, Illinois

Jacob V. DiBattista, BS
Department of Orthopaedic Surgery
Rush University Medical Center
Chicago, Illinois

Melissa G. Goczalk, BFA
Department of Orthopaedic Surgery
Rush University Medical Center
Chicago, Illinois

Brittany E. Haws, MD
Orthopedic Surgery Resident
University of Rochester
Rochester, New York

Fady Y. Hijji, MD
Orthopedic Surgery Resident
Wright State University
Dayton, Ohio

Benjamin Khechen, BA
Research Coordinator
Rush University Medical Center
Chicago, Illinois

Suzanne Labelle, BS
Rush Medical College
Chicago, Illinois

William W. Long, BA
Department of Orthopaedic Surgery
Rush University Medical Center
Chicago, Illinois

Philip K. Louie, MD
Department of Orthopaedic Surgery
Rush University Medical Center
Chicago, Illinois

Catherine Maloney, BS
Department of Orthopaedic Surgery
Rush University Medical Center
Chicago, Illinois

Jonathan Markowitz, BS
Department of Orthopaedic Surgery
Rush University Medical Center
Chicago, Illinois

Dustin H. Massel, BS
Department of Orthopaedic Surgery
Rush University Medical Center
Chicago, Illinois

Benjamin C. Mayo, BA
Department of Orthopaedic Surgery
Rush University Medical Center
Chicago, Illinois

Krishna D. Modi, BS
Department of Orthopaedic Surgery
Rush University Medical Center
Chicago, Illinois

Ankur S. Narain, MD
Orthopedic Surgery Resident
University of Massachusetts
Boston, Massachusetts

Dil V. Patel, BS
Research Coordinator
Rush University Medical Center
Chicago, Illinois

Lauren M. Sadowsky, BA
Rush Medical College
Rush University
Chicago, Illinois

Kern Singh, MD
Professor
Department of Orthopaedic Surgery
Co–Director, Minimally Invasive Spine
    Institute
Rush University Medical Center
Chicago, Illinois

Antonios Varelas, BA
Department of Orthopaedic Surgery
Rush University Medical Center
Chicago, Illinois

# 1 Neuroanatomy and Physiology

*Jacob V. DiBattista, Ankur S. Narain, Fady Y. Hijji, Philip K. Louie, Daniel D. Bohl, and Kern Singh*

## 1.1 Neuron Anatomy

- Basic components (**Table 1.1, Fig. 1.1**).
- Synaptic junction and signal transmission:
  - Mechanism of basic chemical synapses (**Fig. 1.3**).
    - Action potential (depolarization) reaches terminal branch of the presynaptic neuron.
    - N-type $Ca^{2+}$ channels open, $Ca^{2+}$ influx.
      - *Associated pathologies:* Lambert–Eaton myasthenic syndrome.
    - $Ca^{2+}$ facilitates vesicle docking, neurotransmitter released into synaptic cleft.
      - *Associated pathologies:* botulism, tetanus (lockjaw).
    - Neurotransmitter binds neurotransmitter receptor (postsynaptic neuron).
      - *Associated pathologies:* myasthenia gravis.
    - Depending on its function, the neurotransmitter receptor creates either an excitatory postsynaptic potential (EPSP) or an inhibitory postsynaptic potential (IPSP).

Table 1.1 Basic anatomy of the neuron

| Component | Function |
| --- | --- |
| Dendrites | Receive signals from other neurons for transfer toward the cell body |
| Cell body (soma) | Contains cell nucleus. Site of protein and ATP production |
| Axon hillock | Portion of cell body that connects to axon. Final site of action potential summation (trigger zone) |
| Axon | Carries action potential from cell body to terminal branches |
| Myelin sheath | Fatty insulating layer around axon that facilitates action potential through saltatory conduction. <br> • Oligodendrocytes myelinate neurons of the central nervous system (CNS). A single oligodendrocyte myelinates multiple neurons (**Fig. 1.2a**). <br> • Schwann's cells myelinate neurons of the peripheral nervous system (PNS). Multiple Schwann's cells myelinate a single neuron (**Fig. 1.2b**). |
| Nodes of Ranvier | Occasional interruptions in the myelin sheath that expose the axonal membrane. Contain a high density of voltage-gated $Na^+$ and $K^+$ channels and $Na^+/K^+$ ATPases, which act to regenerate the action potential. |
| Terminal branches (boutons) of axon | Branched terminal portion of an axon. Site of neurotransmitter release into the synaptic cleft. Often referred to as the presynaptic terminal. |

1

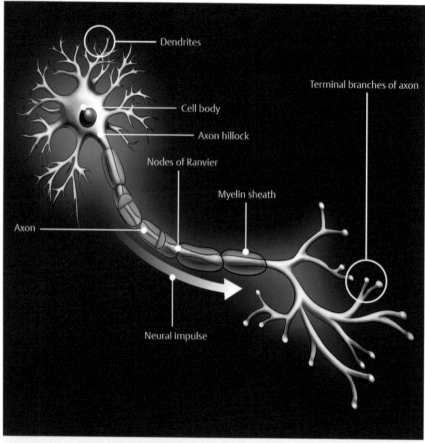

**Fig. 1.1** Basic components of the neuron.

- EPSPs depolarize the postsynaptic neuron and increase the probability of action potential formation.
- IPSPs either hyperpolarize or resist depolarization of the postsynaptic neuron and decrease the probability of action potential formation.
  - The potentials across all dendrites are integrated in the cell body and axon hillock, determining whether or not an action potential will fire in the postsynaptic neuron.
  - A variety of mechanisms, including enzymatic degradation (i.e., acetylcholine) and presynaptic reuptake (i.e., serotonin), remove neurotransmitters from the synaptic cleft to end the postsynaptic stimulus.
- Neuromuscular junction:
  - Specialized chemical synapse between motor neuron and muscle fiber.
  - Cholinergic synapse containing mainly nicotinic acetylcholine receptors.
  - Nerve impulse results in contraction of muscle fiber(s).

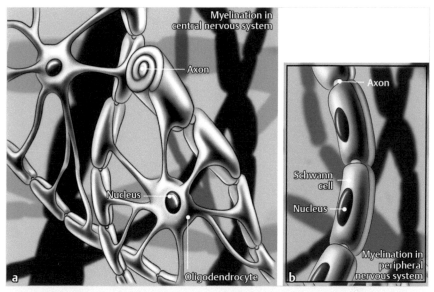

**Fig. 1.2 (a)** Oligodendrocyte (central nervous system). **(b)** Schwann's cell (peripheral nervous system).

- Motor unit:
  - A *single* motor neuron and all muscle fibers that it innervates.
    - A small motor unit contains three to six muscle fibers and controls muscles of fine control.
    - A large motor unit contains 100 to 1,000 muscle fibers and controls muscles of crude control and strength (i.e., biceps, quadriceps).
  - All muscle fibers of a single motor unit are of the same fiber type (types 1, 2a, and 2b).
- Neuron types (**Table 1.2**).
- Nerve fiber organization (**Table 1.3, Fig. 1.4**).
- Nervous system organization (**Fig. 1.5**).
- Afferent and efferent nerves (**Table 1.4, Fig. 1.6**):
  - Afferent nerve fibers carry sensory information and arrive at the spinal cord through dorsal roots.
  - Efferent nerve fibers carry motor information and exit the spinal cord through ventral roots.
  - Efferent motor neurons (**Table 1.5, Fig. 1.7**):
    - Upper motor neurons (UMNs)
      - Cell bodies originate within the primary motor cortex or brainstem nuclei.
      - Convey motor information by synapsing with lower motor neurons (LMNs, or interneurons) in the brainstem or spinal cord.

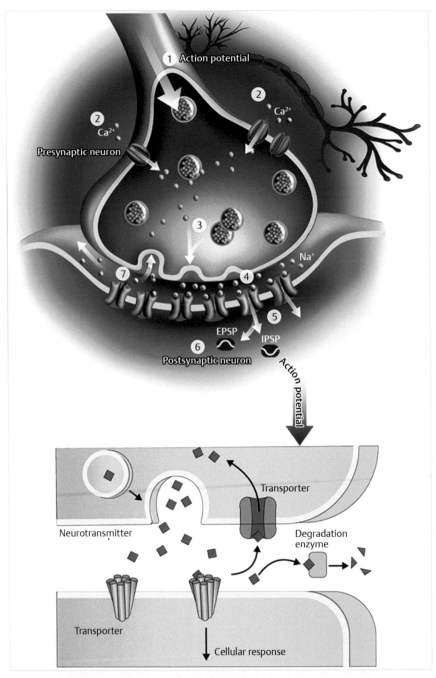

**Fig. 1.3** Synaptic transmission at a chemical synapse.

**Table 1.2** Basic neuron types

| Type | Image | Description | Examples |
|---|---|---|---|
| Pseudounipolar | Dendrites, Initial segment, Axon, Cell body, Axon, Synaptic terminals | A single axon split into two branches with an *adjacent* cell body:<br>• *Peripheral branch*: periphery to cell body (contains dendrites)<br>• *Central branch*: cell body to spinal cord (contains synaptic terminals)<br>Transmits sensory information from the periphery to the CNS | • Sensory neurons of dorsal root ganglia<br>• Sensory ganglia of cranial nerves V, VII, IX, and X |
| Bipolar | Dendrites, Cell body, Axon, Synaptic terminals | Cell body centrally located between a:<br>• *Dendrite:* transmits signals toward cell body<br>• *Axon:* transmits signals away from cell body<br>Specialized sensory neurons for the transmission of special senses (i.e., vision, hearing) | • Bipolar cells, ganglion cells, horizontal cells, and amacrine cells of the retina<br>• Cochlear and vestibular ganglia of the inner ear |
| Multipolar | Dendrites, Cell body, Axon, Synaptic terminals | Cell body contains multiple dendrites and a single axon<br>Able to receive and integrate abundant nerve impulses | • Motor neurons (ventral horn of spinal cord)<br>• Interneurons (spinal cord gray matter)<br>• Purkinje's cells (cerebellum)<br>• Pyramidal cells (cerebral cortex) |

Abbreviation: CNS, central nervous system.

**Table 1.3** Hierarchical organization of nerve fibers

| Component | Covering |
|---|---|
| Deep | |
| Axon (of individual neuron) | Endoneurium |
| Fascicle (bundle of axons) | Perineurium |
| Nerve (bundle of fascicles) | Epineurium |
| Superficial | |

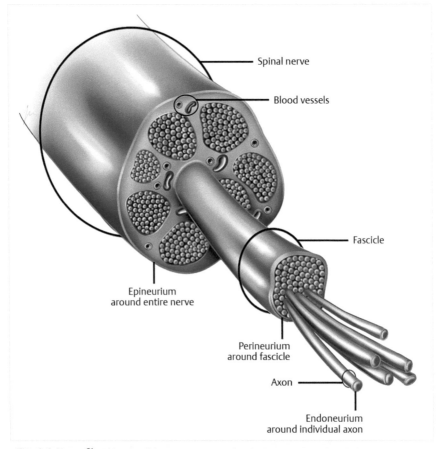

**Fig. 1.4** Nerve fiber structure.

- ○ LMNs:
  - ▪ Cell bodies originate in brainstem nuclei or the ventral horn of spinal cord gray matter.
  - ▪ Convey motor information from UMNs by synapsing with skeletal muscle in the periphery via neuromuscular junctions.
  - Afferent sensory receptors (**Table 1.6**).
  - Afferent sensory neurons (**Table 1.7**).
- Reflex arcs (**Table 1.8**):
  - General principles:
    - ○ A reflex arc is a neural pathway that controls a reflex action.
    - ○ It involves the spinal cord only, allowing for a fast, subconscious response.
    - ○ Sensory information is processed by the brain *after* the reflex has occurred.

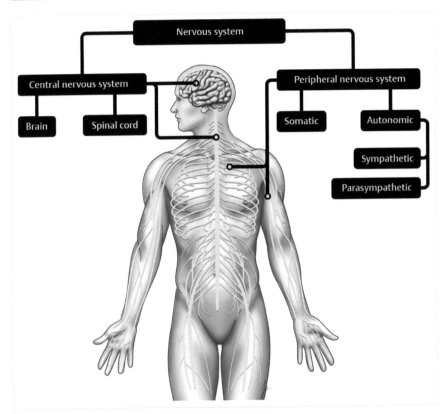

**Fig. 1.5** Summary of central and peripheral nervous systems.

**Table 1.4** Afferent and efferent nerve organization

| Type | Root | Cell body location | Information conveyed |
|---|---|---|---|
| Afferent: | Dorsal | Dorsal root ganglion | Sensory |
| General somatic afferent (GSA) | | | *Skin, muscles, tendons, joints* |
| General visceral afferent (GVA) | | | *Visceral organs* |
| Efferent: | Ventral | Spinal cord gray matter | Motor |
| General somatic efferent (GSE) | | *Ventral horn* | *Skeletal muscle* |
| General visceral efferent (GVE) | | *Lateral horn* | *Smooth and cardiac muscle, glands* |

Note: In spinal nerves and dorsal and ventral rami, GSA, GVA, GSE, and GVE fibers are mixed.

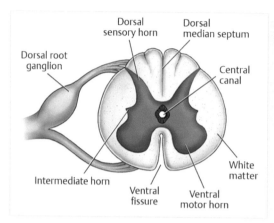

**Fig. 1.6** Components of spinal nerves. (Reproduced with permission from Baaj AA, Mummaneni PV, Uribe JS, Vaccaro AR, Greenberg MS, eds. Handbook of Spine Surgery. 2nd ed. New York, NY: Thieme; 2016.)

**Table 1.5** General signs of upper motor neuron and lower motor neuron lesions

| Clinical sign | Upper motor neuron lesion presentation | | Lower motor neuron lesion presentation |
| --- | --- | --- | --- |
| | Acute | Chronic | |
| Weakness | Yes | Yes | Yes |
| Atrophy | No | Some | Severe |
| Tone/paralysis | Decreased/flaccid | Increased/spastic | Decreased |
| Fasciculations | No[a] | No[a] | Yes |
| Reflexes | Decreased | Increased | Decreased |
| Babinski's sign[b] | No | Yes | No |

[a]May see slight fasciculations at spinal level of UMN lesions due to partial damage of LMN cell bodies in the ventral horn.
[b]Babinski's sign is considered normal response in children younger than 1 year.

- Types:
  - Monosynaptic: contains two neurons (sensory and motor) with a single chemical synapse (**Fig. 1.9**):
    - That is, patellar reflex, Achilles reflex.
  - Polysynaptic: contains one or more interneurons that connect a sensory neuron to a motor neuron:
    - Represents the majority of reflex arcs.
    - Allows for higher order processing and control.
    - That is, pain withdrawal reflex.
  - Somatic: affects skeletal muscle.
  - Autonomic: affects internal viscera.
- Components:
  - Stimulus (muscle stretch, pain, temperature, stretch, etc.).
  - Sensory receptor (muscle spindle, free nerve ending, etc.).

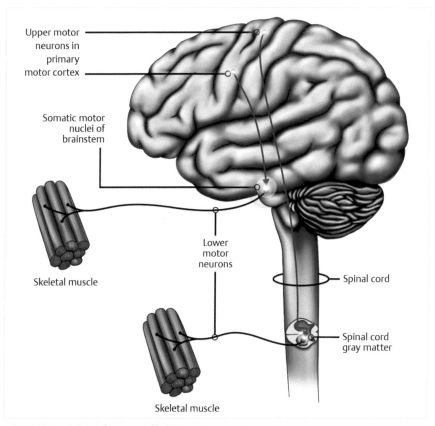

**Fig. 1.7** Depiction of upper and lower motor neurons.

- Afferent pathway: sensory neuron (dorsal root ganglia).
- Interneuron(s) (dorsal horn):
  - Polysynaptic reflex arcs only.
- Efferent pathway: motor neuron (ventral horn).
- Skeletal muscle:
  - Effector response → muscle contraction.
- Inhibitory interneurons:
  - Activated by sensory neurons of a reflex arc.
  - Inhibit LMNs that act on antagonistic muscle groups:
    - That is, during biceps reflex, inhibitory interneurons will cause the triceps to relax.
- UMN effects:
  - Inhibits the magnitude of LMN responses in a reflex arc:
    - This is a conscious process, and is the basis of the Jendrassik maneuver:

**Table 1.6** Sensory receptor types

| Receptor type | Modality | Adaption rate | Fiber class |
|---|---|---|---|
| Cutaneous mechanoreceptors | | | |
| Meissner's corpuscle | Touch (superficial) | Rapid | II |
| Merkel's cell | Touch (superficial) | Slow | II |
| Hair follicle receptor | Touch, vibration | Rapid and slow | II |
| Pacinian corpuscle | Touch (deep), vibration | Rapid | II |
| Ruffini's ending | Touch (deep), stretch, proprioception | Very slow | II |
| Stretch receptors | | | |
| Muscle spindle | | | |
| Nuclear bag fibers | Proprioception (muscle stretch) | Slow | I |
| Nuclear chain fibers | Proprioception (muscle tone) | Slow | II |
| Golgi's tendon organ | Proprioception (muscle tension) | Slow | I |
| Pain and temperature receptors | | | |
| Free nerve endings | Nociception (fast) | – | III |
|  | Nociception (slow) | – | IV |
|  | Temperature (cool) | – | III |
|  | Temperature (warm) | – | IV |

**Table 1.7** Types of sensory neuron fibers

| Sensory fiber type | Myelinated | Sensory modality | Sensory receptor |
|---|---|---|---|
| A-α[a] | Yes | Proprioception | Muscle spindle<br>Golgi's tendon organ |
| A-β | Yes | Proprioception<br>Superficial touch<br>Touch, vibration<br>Deep touch, vibration<br>Deep touch, stretch | Muscle spindle<br>Meissner's corpuscle<br>Merkel's cell<br>Hair follicle receptor<br>Pacinian corpuscle<br>Ruffini's ending |
| A-δ | Yes | Nociception (fast)<br>Temperature (cool) | Free nerve endings<br>Free nerve endings |
| C[b] | No | Nociception (slow)<br>Temperature (warm) | Free nerve endings<br>Free nerve endings |

[a]A-α fibers have the lowest threshold for stimulation.
[b]C fibers have the highest threshold for stimulation.

**Table 1.8** Commonly tested deep tendon reflexes

| Deep tendon reflex | Spinal cord level tested |
| --- | --- |
| Biceps reflex | C5–C6 |
| Brachioradialis reflex | C6 |
| Triceps reflex | C6–C8 |
| Patellar reflex (knee jerk) | L2–L4 |
| Achilles reflex (ankle jerk) | S1–S2 |

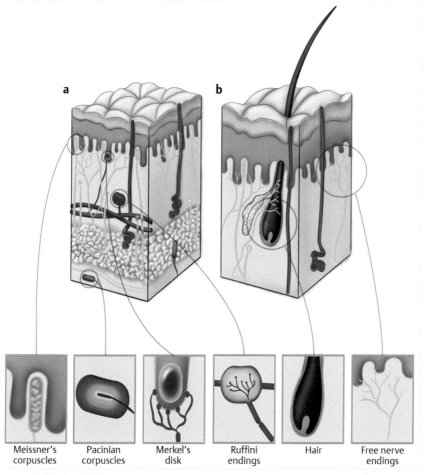

Meissner's corpuscles | Pacinian corpuscles | Merkel's disk | Ruffini endings | Hair | Free nerve endings

**Fig. 1.8 (a)** Location of different sensory receptor types in skin tissue. **(b)** Location of Type I and Type II fibers within muscle tissue.

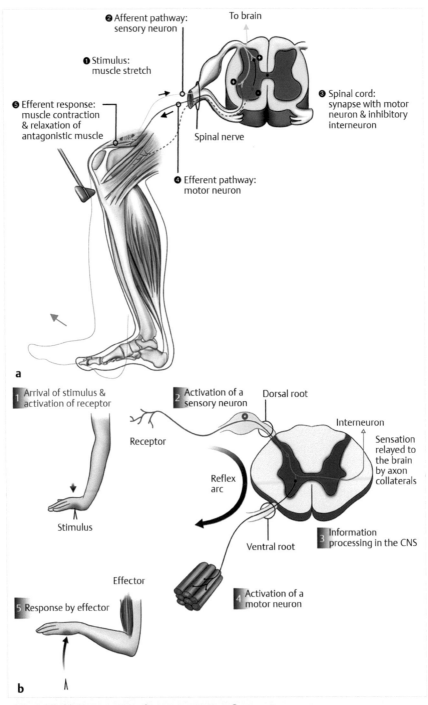

**❷ Afferent pathway:**
sensory neuron

**To brain**

**❶ Stimulus:**
muscle stretch

**❺ Efferent response:**
muscle contraction
& relaxation of
antagonistic muscle

**❸ Spinal cord:**
synapse with motor
neuron & inhibitory
interneuron

Spinal nerve

**❹ Efferent pathway:**
motor neuron

**a**

**1** Arrival of stimulus &
activation of receptor

**2** Activation of a
sensory neuron

Dorsal root

Interneuron

Receptor

Sensation
relayed to
the brain
by axon
collaterals

Reflex
arc

Stimulus

Information
**3** processing in the CNS

Ventral root

Effector

**5** Response by effector

**4** Activation of a
motor neuron

**b**

**Fig. 1.9 (a,b)** Components of a monosynaptic reflex arc.

❖ Useful to determine the effect of UMNs on clinically observed hyporeflexia.
❖ Can reduce the effect of UMNs on a reflex arc by having a patient clench their teeth and hold their interlocked fingers in a hooklike configuration.
❖ These maneuvers reduce the conscious activity of UMNs by providing a distraction.

- Lesions
  ◦ UMN lesions → hyperreflexia due to loss of inhibition.
  ◦ LMN lesions → hyporeflexia due to loss of effector response.

## Suggested Readings

1. Haines DE. Fundamental Neuroscience for Basic and Clinical Applications. 4th ed. Philadelphia, PA: Churchill Livingstone/Elsevier; 2013
2. Haines DE. Neuroanatomy in Clinical Context: An Atlas of Structures, Sections, and Systems. 9th ed. Baltimore, MD: Lippincott, Williams, and Wilkins; 2014
3. Drake RL, Vogl AW, Mitchell AW. Gray's Anatomy for Students. 2nd ed. Philadelphia, PA: Churchill Livingstone; 2014
4. Gilroy AM, MacPherson BR, Ross LM, Schuenke M, Schulte E, Schumacher U. Atlas of Anatomy. 2nd ed. New York, NY: Thieme; 2012
5. Martini FH, Timmons MJ, Tallitsch RB. Human Anatomy. 8th ed. Boston, MA: Pearson; 2014

# 2 General Spine Anatomy and Long Tract Pathways

*Jacob V. DiBattista, Ankur S. Narain, Fady Y. Hijji, Philip K. Louie, Daniel D. Bohl, and Kern Singh*

## 2.1 Topographical Anatomy

### 2.1.1 General Vertebral Column Anatomy

• Overview of the vertebral column (**Table 2.1, Fig. 2.1**).
• Column classification:
  – Vertebral column divided into three anatomical classifications (**Table 2.2, Fig. 2.2**).
  – Moderate reliability for determining clinical degree of stability.
• Surface landmarks (**Table 2.3, Fig. 2.3**).

### 2.1.2 General Spinal Cord Anatomy

• Vertebral canal:
  – Spans from foramen magnum (cranial) to the sacral hiatus (caudal).
  – Formed by the vertebral foramina of each vertebra.
  – Contents (**Table 2.4, Fig. 2.4**).
• Spinal cord regions and spinal nerves:
  – Five divisions and 31 spinal nerves (**Fig. 2.5**):
    ◦ Cervical: C1–C8 spinal nerves.
    ◦ Thoracic: T1–T12 spinal nerves.

**Table 2.1** Regions of the vertebral column

| Region | Vertebral levels | Curvature[a] | Function |
|---|---|---|---|
| Cervical | C1–C7 | Lordosis, 20–40 degrees | Supports and moves head Transmits spinal cord and vertebral vessels between head and neck |
| Thoracic | T1–T12 | Kyphosis, 20–40 degrees | Supports and protects thorax |
| Lumbar | L1–L5 | Lordosis, 40–60 degrees | Supports abdomen |
| Sacral | S1–S5 (fused) | Kyphosis, fused | Transmits weight to lower limbs through the pelvic bones Forms boundary and framework of posterior pelvis |
| Coccyx | Co | Kyphosis | Vestigial, no apparent function |

[a]Kyphosis: concave anteriorly and convex posteriorly. Lordosis: convex anteriorly and concave posteriorly.

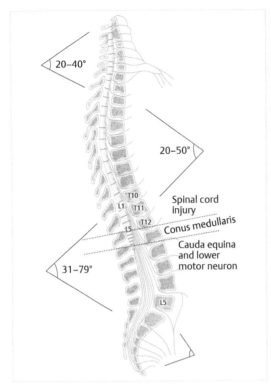

**Fig. 2.1** Vertebral column. (Reproduced with permission from An HS, Singh K, eds. Synopsis of Spine Surgery. 3rd ed. New York, NY: Thieme; 2016.)

**Table 2.2** Column classification

| Classification | Anterior boundary | Posterior boundary |
|---|---|---|
| Anterior column | Anterior longitudinal ligament (ALL) | Anterior two-thirds of vertebral body and intervertebral disk |
| Middle column | Posterior one-third of vertebral body and intervertebral disk | Posterior longitudinal ligament (PLL) |
| Posterior column | Immediately posterior to PLL | Ligamentum nuchae (C1–C7) or supraspinous ligament (inferior to C7) |

- ○ Lumbar: L1–L5 spinal nerves.
- ○ Sacral: S1–S5 spinal nerves.
- ○ Coccyx: coccygeal nerve.
- Spinal nerves exit vertebral canal through intervertebral foramina.
- Spinal nerve numbering:
  - ○ C1–C7 spinal nerves exit *above* their respective vertebrae.
  - ○ C8 spinal nerve exits *below* C7 vertebrae (C7/T1 intervertebral foramen).
  - ○ All remaining spinal nerves exit *below* their respective vertebrae.

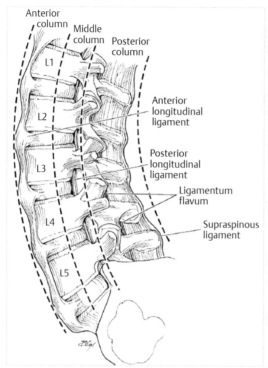

Anterior column
Middle column
Posterior column
L1
L2
L3
L4
L5

Anterior longitudinal ligament

Posterior longitudinal ligament

Ligamentum flavum

Supraspinous ligament

**Fig. 2.2** Column classification. (Reproduced with permission from Baaj AA, Mummaneni PV, Uribe JS, Vaccaro AR, Greenberg MS, eds. Handbook of Spine Surgery. 2nd ed. New York, NY: Thieme; 2016.)

**Table 2.3** Palpable surface landmarks and association with vertebral level

| | Anterior | | Posterior |
|---|---|---|---|
| Vertebral level | Surface landmark | Vertebral level | Surface landmark |
| C2/C3 | Body of mandible | C7 | Most prominent |
| T2/T3 | Jugular notch | T3 | Spine of scapula (medial portion) |
| T9/T10 | Xiphoid process | T7 | Inferior tip of scapula |
| L3/L4 | Umbilicus | L4 | Superior aspect of iliac crests |
| S1 | Anterior superior iliac spine (ASIS) | S2 | Posterior superior iliac spine (PSIS) |

• General features of the spinal cord:
  – Adult spinal cord is two-thirds the length of the vertebral column:
    ◦ Origin: medulla (brainstem) at the foramen magnum.
    ◦ Termination: conus medullaris (L2).
  – Thecal sac comprises a dura-surrounded sac that extends from the spinal cord and contains cerebrospinal fluid (CSF), nerve roots, and the cauda equina.
  – Features (**Table 2.5, Figs. 2.5, 2.6**).

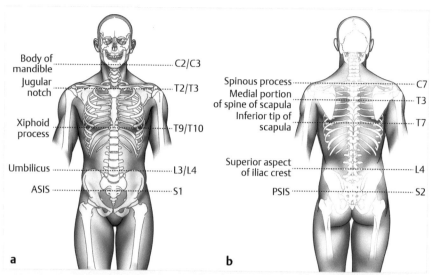

**Fig. 2.3** Palpable surface landmarks to determine vertebral level. **(a)** Anterior. **(b)** Posterior.

**Table 2.4** Contents of the vertebral canal

| Structure | Description |
| --- | --- |
| *Superficial* | |
| Extradural (epidural) space | Contains adipose tissue and internal vertebral venous plexus |
| Internal vertebral venous plexus (anterior and posterior divisions) | Drains spinal cord and connects with external vertebral plexus. Lack of valves can lead to bidirectional blood flow |
| Meningeal layers | |
| • Dura mater (most superficial) | Composed of fibrous tissue. Continuous with the epineurium of spinal nerves |
| Subdural space | Potential space between dura and arachnoid mater that can open secondary to trauma (i.e., subdural hematoma) |
| • Arachnoid mater (middle) | Adherent to dura mater. Avascular and translucent |
| Subarachnoid space | Between arachnoid and pia mater. Contains cerebrospinal fluid (CSF) |
| • Pia mater (deepest) | Composed of thin fibrous tissue. Impermeable to CSF |
| Denticulate ligaments | Reflections of pia mater that attach to the arachnoid and dura mater. 21 pairs, spanning craniovertebral junction to T12, provide stability to the spinal cord |
| Spinal cord | |
| *Deep* | |

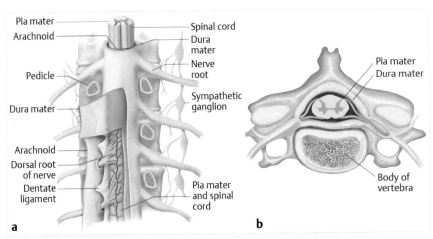

**Fig. 2.4 (a,b)** Contents of the vertebral canal. (Reproduced with permission from Baaj AA, Mummaneni PV, Uribe JS, Vaccaro AR, Greenberg MS, eds. Handbook of Spine Surgery. 2nd ed. New York, NY: Thieme; 2016.)

- Spinal cord anatomy (**Tables 2.6–2.7**).
- Regional variation in spinal cord white and gray matter composition (**Figs. 2.7, 2.8**):
  - Cervical region:
    - Abundant gray matter for innervation of upper extremities.
    - Region of most abundant white matter.
    - Presence of both the fasciculus gracilis and cuneatus.
  - Thoracic region:
    - Reduced size of gray matter (no innervation to extremities).
    - Less white matter than cervical region.
    - Intermediolateral (IML) cell column:
      - Small outpocketing of gray matter from lateral horn containing cell bodies of preganglionic sympathetic neurons.
    - Fasciculus cuneatus only present superior to T6, while fasciculus gracilis is present over the entire length.
  - Lumbar region:
    - Abundant gray matter for innervation of lower extremities.
    - Less white matter than superior regions.
    - Presence of the fasciculus gracilis only.
    - Presence of cauda equina.
  - Sacral region:
    - Comparatively little white or gray matter.
    - Contains an IML cell column:
      - Cell bodies of parasympathetic preganglionic neurons.
    - Presence of cauda equina.

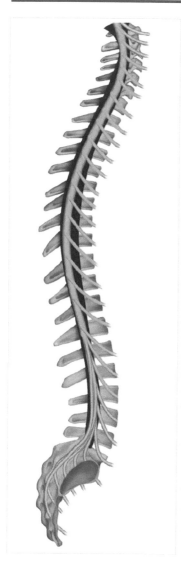

**Fig. 2.5** Spinal cord regions, features, and spinal nerve. (Reproduced with permission from Albert TJ, Vaccaro, AR, eds. Physical Examination of the Spine. 2nd ed. New York, NY: Thieme; 2016.)

## 2.2  Long Tract Pathways

- Descending tracts (motor information; **Tables 2.8, 2.9, Fig. 2.9**).
- Ascending tracts (sensory information; **Tables 2.10, 2.11**).

**Table 2.5**  General features of the spinal cord

| Feature and vertebral level | Description |
| --- | --- |
| Cervical enlargement (C4–T1) | Overabundance of nerve fibers for the innervation of upper extremities |
| Lumbosacral enlargement (L1–L3) | Overabundance of nerve fibers for the innervation of lower extremities |
| Cauda equina (T12/L1–Co) | Collection of lumbar, sacral, and coccygeal nerve roots that arise from the conus medullaris<br>Travel inferiorly within vertebral canal to exit at their respective vertebral levels |
| Termination of dural sac (S2) | Termination of dura mater |
| Filum terminale | Continuation of pia mater from conus medullaris (L2) to the coccyx. Helps anchor spinal cord in place |
| Internum (L2–S2) | Filum terminale within the dural sac |
| Externum (S2–Co) | Filum terminale outside the dural sac |

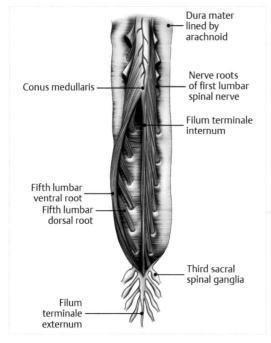

Dura mater lined by arachnoid

Conus medullaris

Nerve roots of first lumbar spinal nerve

Filum terminale internum

Fifth lumbar ventral root

Fifth lumbar dorsal root

Third sacral spinal ganglia

Filum terminale externum

**Fig. 2.6**  Terminal ending of the spinal cord.

**Table 2.6** Spinal cord anatomy: surface structures

| Structure | Function |
|---|---|
| Root | |
| Ventral | Carries **motor** information from the spinal cord. Contains general somatic efferent (GSE) and general visceral efferent (GVE) fibers |
| Dorsal | Carries **sensory** information to the spinal cord. Contains general somatic afferent (GSA) and general visceral afferent (GVA) fibers |
| Rootlet | |
| Ventral | Branched portion of ventral root that attaches to spinal cord |
| Dorsal | Branched potion of dorsal root that attaches to spinal cord |
| Dorsal root ganglion | Site of GSA and GVA neuron cell bodies |
| Spinal nerve | Aggregation of ventral and dorsal roots (GSA, GVA, GSE, and GVE fibers). 31 pairs, which exit vertebral canal at intervertebral foramina |
| Ramus | |
| Ventral | Anterior division of a spinal nerve. Innervates the ventral trunk and upper and lower limbs. Much larger than the dorsal mini |
| Dorsal | Posterior division of a spinal nerve. Most levels divide into medial and lateral branches to innervate skin and muscles of back (dorsal trunk) |
| Meningeal branches | Branch from spinal nerve prior to rami. Re-enter intervertebral foramen to innervate vertebrae and vertebral canal structures |
| Anterior median fissure | Runs length of ventral spinal cord, dividing it into right and left halves. Creates a groove where the anterior spinal artery lies |
| Anterolateral sulcus | Site where ventral rootlets exit the spinal cord |
| Posterior median sulcus | Runs length of dorsal spinal cord, dividing it into right and left halves. Less prominent than anterior median sulcus |
| Posterior intermediate sulcus | Small furrow that separates the fasciculus gracilis (medial) from the fasciculus cuneatus (lateral). Only located superior to T6 |
| Posterolateral sulcus | Site where dorsal rootlets enter the spinal cord |

# 2.3 Intervertebral Disk Anatomy (Fig. 2.10)

• Description:
  - Nonsynovial (symphysis) joint located between vertebral bodies:
    ◦ Layer of hyaline cartilage separates the disk and vertebral body (end plates).
• Composition:
  - Fibrocartilaginous.
  - Nucleus pulposus: inner core, remnant of the embryological notochord:
    ◦ Composed of type II collagen.
  - Annulus fibrosus: outer ring arranged in lamellar fashion:
    ◦ Composed of type I collagen.

**Table 2.7** Spinal cord anatomy: cross section

| White matter: myelinated neurons. Contains ascending and descending tracts (pathways). | |
|---|---|
| Structure[a] | Function (tracts) |
| Anterior funiculus | Ascending: anterior spinothalamic<br>Descending: anterior corticospinal, medial reticulospinal, tectospinal, and medial vestibulospinal |
| Lateral funiculus | Ascending: lateral spinothalamic and anterior and posterior spinocerebellar<br>Descending: lateral corticospinal, lateral reticulospinal, rubrospinal, and lateral vestibulospinal |
| Posterior funiculus | Ascending: dorsal column (fasciculus gracilis and cuneatus)<br>Descending: none |
| Anterior white commissure | Site where certain fibers cross in the midline. Located between the anterior median fissure and gray matter commissure. Connects two halves of spinal cord |
| Gray matter: unmyelinated neurons. Contains interneurons and cell bodies. | |
| Structure | Function |
| Ventral horn | Site of GSE cell bodies (lower motor neurons) |
| Lateral horn | Site of GVE (autonomic) cell bodies |
| Dorsal horn | Site of interneuron cell bodies (receive GSA and GVA fibers) |
| Gray commissure | Surrounds central canal. Connects two halves of spinal cord |
| Other structures | |
| Structure | Function |
| Central canal | Cerebrospinal fluid–filled space within the center of the spinal cord. Continuous with the ventricular system of the brain. Gradually occludes with age |

[a]A fasciculus refers to a bundle of parallel axons in the central nervous system (carry same information/modality), while a funiculus refers to a grouping of fasciculi. Both are located within spinal cord white matter.

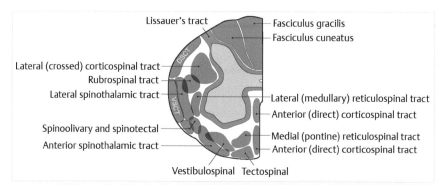

**Fig. 2.7** Divisions of spinal cord white matter and gray matter. (Reproduced with permission from Fehlings MG, Vaccaro AR, Maxwell Boakye M, Rossignol S, Ditunno DF, Burns AS, eds. Essentials of Spinal Cord Injury: Basic Research to Clinical Practice. New York, NY: Thieme; 2012.)

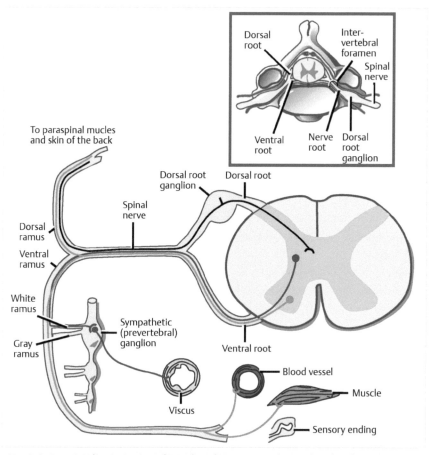

**Fig. 2.8** Functional organization of spinal cord gray matter. (Reproduced with permission from Albertstone CD, Benzel EC, Najm IM, Steinmetz M, eds. Anatomic Basis of Neurologic Diagnosis. New York, NY: Thieme; 2009.)

- Mechanics:
  - Allows limited movement and holds vertebrae in close association.
  - Help resist compression of the vertebral column.
- Anatomy:
  - Twenty-three pairs of disks in the vertebral column:
    - First intervertebral disk: C2/C3.
    - Last functional intervertebral disk: L5/S1.

**Table 2.8** Overview of the descending (motor) tracts

| | | |
|---|---|---|
| *Pyramidal tracts:* UMN fibers that travel from the cerebral cortex to the spinal cord. Control voluntary movement by acting directly (or indirectly via interneurons) on lower motor neuron (LMN) cell bodies of the ventral horn. | | |

| Tract | Location | |
|---|---|---|
| | Spinal cord white matter | Spinal cord region |
| Corticospinal | | |
| Anterior | Anterior funiculus | Entire length |
| Lateral | Lateral funiculus | Entire length |

| | | |
|---|---|---|
| *Extrapyramidal tracts:* upper motor neuron (UMN) fibers that travel from brainstem areas to the spinal cord. Control involuntary movements by modulating and regulating LMN cell bodies of the ventral horn (i.e., posture, balance, etc.). | | |

| Tract | Location | |
|---|---|---|
| | Spinal cord white matter | Spinal cord region |
| Reticulospinal | | |
| Medial | Anterior funiculus | Entire length |
| Lateral | Lateral funiculus | Entire length |
| Rubrospinal | Lateral funiculus | Cervical/upper thoracic only |
| Tectospinal | Anterior funiculus | Cervical only |
| Vestibulospinal | | |
| Medial | Anterior funiculus | Cervical only |
| Lateral | Lateral funiculus | Entire length |

# 2.4 Dermatomes

• Dermatome:
  - Distinct area of skin supplied by a single spinal cord level.
  - That is, pain sensation from a pinprick on the third finger is carried through the median nerve and enters the spinal cord at C7.
• Radiating pain:
  - Pain that migrates from the origin of the painful stimulus; can be cutaneous or deep.
  - That is, sciatica is caused by L5 spinal nerve entrapment, leading to lower back pain that radiates down the thigh to the leg and foot.
• Referred pain:
  - Pain perceived at a different site than origin of the painful stimulus.
  - Follows dermatomal pattern (based on autonomics).
  - That is, a myocardial infarction often causes pain in the left shoulder, neck, and back because general visceral afferent (GVA) fibers from the heart are of the same spinal level and dermatome as those cutaneous areas.

**Table 2.9** Descending (motor) tract pathway details

| Tract | Function | Pathway | | Site of decussation |
| --- | --- | --- | --- | --- |
| | | Origin | Final destination | |
| **Corticospinal** | | | | |
| Anterior[a] | Control of proximal muscles (trunk and neck) | Cerebral cortex (precentral gyrus) | Lower motor neuron (LMN) cell bodies | Some in anterior white commissure, at level of synapse (bilateral innervation) |
| Lateral | Control of fine movement in (primarily) distal flexor muscles | Cerebral cortex (precentral gyrus) | LMN cell bodies | Caudal medulla (contralateral innervation) |
| **Reticulospinal** | | | | |
| Medial | Regulation of voluntary movement in (primarily) extensors of limbs and trunk | Pontine reticular formation | Interneurons (dorsal horn) | None (ipsilateral innervation) |
| Lateral | Regulation of voluntary movement in (primarily) flexors of limbs | Medullary reticular formation | Interneurons (dorsal horn) | Some in caudal medulla (bilateral innervation) |
| Rubrospinal | Facilitation of voluntary movement in flexors of upper limbs. Inhibition of voluntary movement in extensors of upper limbs. Important for balance | Red nucleus (midbrain) | Interneurons and LMN cell bodies | Midbrain (contralateral innervation) |
| Tectospinal | Reflex movement of head and neck due to visual stimuli | Superior colliculus (midbrain) | Interneurons and LMN cell bodies | Midbrain (contralateral innervation) |
| **Vestibulospinal** | | | | |
| Medial | Maintain upright head positioning in response to vestibular stimuli | Medial vestibular nucleus (medulla) | Interneurons and LMN cell bodies | Some in caudal medulla (bilateral innervation) |
| Lateral | Maintain posture in response to vestibular stimuli | Lateral vestibular nucleus (pons) | LMN cell bodies | None (ipsilateral innervation) |

[a]The anterior corticospinal pathway represents approximately 15% of neurons that do not decussate in the lower medulla (which form the lateral corticospinal pathway).

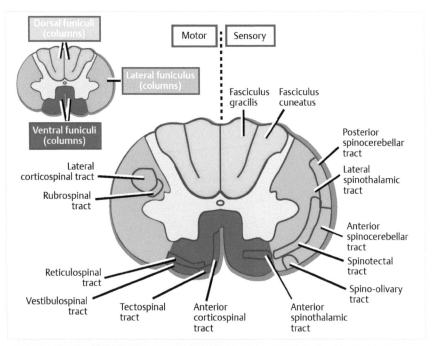

**Fig. 2.9** Descending (motor) and ascending (sensory) tracts. (Reproduced with permission from Albertstone CD, Benzel EC, Najm IM, Steinmetz M, eds. Anatomic Basis of Neurologic Diagnosis. New York, NY: Thieme; 2009.)

**Table 2.10** Overview of the ascending (sensory) tracts

| Tract | Location | |
|---|---|---|
| | Spinal cord white matter | Spinal cord region |
| Dorsal column | | |
| Fasciculus cuneatus | Posterior funiculus | Cranially to T6 only |
| Fasciculus gracilis | Posterior funiculus | Entire length |
| Spinothalamic | | |
| Anterior | Anterior funiculus | Entire length |
| Lateral | Lateral funiculus | Entire length |
| Spinocerebellar | | |
| Anterior | Lateral funiculus | Entire length |
| Posterior | Lateral funiculus | Entire length |

**Table 2.11** Ascending (sensory) tract pathway details

| Tract | Sensory modality | Cell body location and pathway | | | | Site of decussation |
|---|---|---|---|---|---|---|
| | | 1-degree neuron | 2-degree neuron | 3-degree neuron | Terminal destination | |
| Dorsal column | | | | | | |
| Fasciculus gracilis | Conscious proprioception, 2-point discrimination, touch, pressure, and vibration caudal to T6 | Dorsal root ganglia. Ascends within fasciculus gracilis (medial portion of posterior funiculus) | Nucleus gracilis of medulla. Decussates and ascends within medial lemniscus | Ventral posterolateral (VPL) nucleus of thalamus. Ascends within internal capsule | Cerebral cortex (postcentral gyrus) | Lower medulla (contralateral sensation) |
| Fasciculus cuneatus | Conscious proprioception, 2-point discrimination, touch, pressure, and vibration cranial to T6 | Dorsal root ganglia. Ascends within fasciculus cuneatus (lateral portion of posterior funiculus) | Nucleus cuneatus of medulla. Decussates and ascends within medial lemniscus | Same as above | Same as above | Same as above |
| Spinothalamic | | | | | | |
| Anterior | Light touch | Dorsal root ganglia. Either enters dorsal horn at same level or travels 1–2 levels cranially or caudally via Lissauer's tract | Substantia gelatinosa or nucleus proprius of dorsal horn. Decussates via the anterior white commissure and ascends in the anterior funiculus | VPL nucleus of thalamus. Ascends within internal capsule | Cerebral cortex (postcentral gyrus) | Anterior white commissure, at either same spinal level or 1–2 cranially or caudally (contralateral sensation) |
| Lateral | Pain and temperature | Same as above | Same as above, but ascends in the lateral funiculus | Same as above | Same as above | Same as above |

*(Continued)*

Table 2.11 (Continued)

| Tract | Sensory modality | Cell body location and pathway | | | | Site of decussation |
|---|---|---|---|---|---|---|
| | | 1-degree neuron | 2-degree neuron | 3-degree neuron | Terminal destination | |
| Spinocerebellar | | | | | | |
| Anterior | Unconscious proprioception | Dorsal root ganglia. Enters dorsal horn at same level | Nucleus proprius. Decussates via the anterior white commissure and ascends in the lateral funiculus | None | Cerebellum (via superior cerebellar peduncle of midbrain) | Anterior white commissure at same level, then again in the cerebellum (net ipsilateral sensation) |
| Posterior | Unconscious proprioception | Same as above | Nucleus of Clarke. Ascends ipsilaterally in the lateral funiculus | None | Cerebellum (via inferior cerebellar peduncle of midbrain) | None (ipsilateral sensation) |

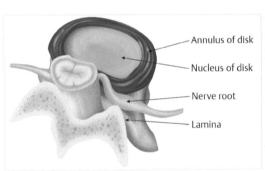

Annulus of disk

Nucleus of disk

Nerve root

Lamina

**Fig. 2.10 (a,b)** Components of the intervertebral disks. (Reproduced with permission from An HS, Singh K, eds. Synopsis of Spine Surgery. 3rd ed. New York, NY: Thieme; 2016.)

## Suggested Readings

1.  Haines DE. Fundamental Neuroscience for Basic and Clinical Applications. 4th ed. Philadelphia, PA: Churchill Livingstone/Elsevier; 2013
2.  Haines DE. Neuroanatomy in Clinical Context: An Atlas of Structures, Sections, and Systems. 9th ed. Baltimore, MD: Lippincott, Williams, and Wilkins; 2014
3.  Drake RL, Vogl AW, Mitchell AW. Gray's Anatomy for Students. 2nd ed. Philadelphia, PA: Churchill Livingstone; 2014
4.  Gilroy AM, MacPherson BR, Ross LM, Schuenke M, Schulte E, Schumacher U. Atlas of Anatomy. 2nd ed. New York, NY: Thieme; 2012
5.  Martini FH, Timmons MJ, Tallitsch RB. Human Anatomy. 8th ed. Boston, MA: Pearson; 2014

# 3 Atlanto-Occipital Anatomy

*Suzanne Labelle, Fady Y. Hijji, Ankur S. Narain, Philip K. Louie, Daniel D. Bohl, and Kern Singh*

## 3.1 Bony Anatomy

### 3.1.1 Occipital Bone (Fig. 3.1)

- External occipital protuberance.
- Superior nuchal line.
- Inferior nuchal line.
- Occipital condyle:
  - Articulate with superior facets of the atlas vertebra.

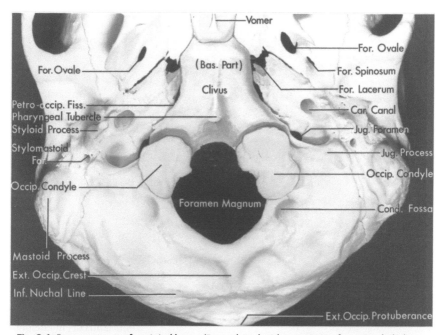

**Fig. 3.1** Bony anatomy of occipital bone. (Reproduced with permission from Bambakidis NC, Dickman CA, Spetzler RF, Sonntag VKH, eds. Surgery of the Craniovertebral Junction. 2nd edition. New York, NY: Thieme; 2012)

## 3.1.2 Atlas: First Cervical Vertebra (C1; Fig. 3.2)

- Foramen magnum:
  - Allows passage of spinal cord.
- Anterior arch:
  - Anterior tubercle.
  - Articular facet for dens on posterior surface.

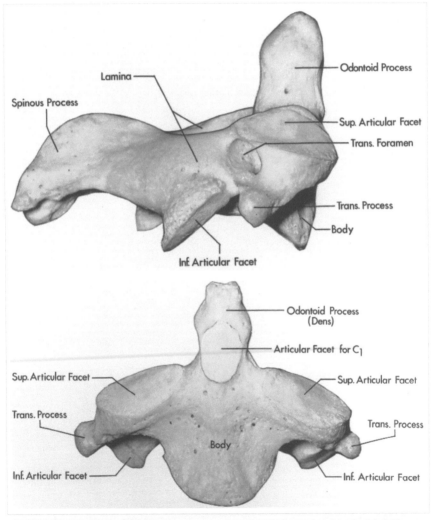

**Fig. 3.2** Bony anatomy of atlas and axis. (Reproduced with permission from Bambakidis NC, Dickman CA, Spetzler RF, Sonntag VKH, eds. Surgery of the Craniovertebral Junction. 2nd edition. New York, NY: Thieme; 2012)

• Posterior arch:
  - Equivalent to lamina of other cervical vertebrae.
  - Posterior tubercle:
    ◦ Equivalent to spinous process.
• Transverse process:
  - Contains transverse foramen:
    ◦ Allows for passage of vertebral artery.
    ◦ Vertically oriented.
• Lateral masses:
  - Equivalent to vertebral body (no formal vertebral body).
  - Contains tubercle for attachment of cruciate ligament.
  - Superior articular surface:
    ◦ Horizontally oriented.
    ◦ Articulates with occipital condyle forming atlanto-occipital joint:
      ▪ Biaxial condyloid synovial joint: fluid-filled articulations involving occipital condyles that allow movement in two planes.
      ▪ Permits flexion and extension; minimal lateral bending and rotation.
  - Inferior articular surface:
    ◦ Horizontally oriented.
    ◦ Articulates with lateral mass of axis forming atlanto-axial joint.

## 3.1.3  Axis: Second Cervical Vertebra (C2; Fig. 3.2)

• Dens:
  - Unique to only C2.
  - Anterior articular facet:
    ◦ Articulates with anterior arch of atlas.
    ◦ Forms median pivot joint (**Fig. 3.3**).
  - Posterior articular facet:
    ◦ Serves as articulating surface for the transverse ligament of the cruciate ligament:
      ▪ Prevents subluxation between C1 and C2.

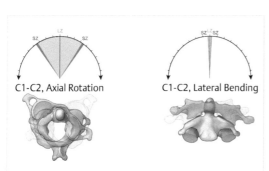

**Fig. 3.3** Atlantoaxial joint side-to-side rotation. (Reproduced with permission from Bambakidis NC, Dickman CA, Spetzler RF, Sonntag VKH, eds. Surgery of the Craniovertebral Junction. 2nd edition. New York, NY: Thieme; 2012)

  - Small vertebral body beneath dens:
    ◦ Small pedicles attaching to lateral masses.
- Transverse process:
  - Contains transverse foramen:
    ◦ Vertebral artery exits here:
      ▪ Makes a 45-degree turn and re-enters cervical spine at transverse foramen of C1.
- Spinous process:
  - Small and bifid.
- Lateral masses:
  - Superior articular facet:
    ◦ Horizontally oriented.
    ◦ Articulates with atlas forming atlantoaxial joint:
      ▪ Uniaxial synovial joint: fluid-filled joint that allows movement in one plane.
      ▪ Plane joints between both superior articular facets of axis and corresponding inferior articular facets of atlas.
      ▪ Median pivot joint between dens and anterior arch of atlas.
      ▪ Permits side-to-side head rotation (50% of cervical rotation).
      ▪ Permits small degree of flexion/extension (10 of 110 degrees of the cervical spine).
  - Inferior articular facet:
    ◦ Horizontally oriented.
    ◦ Articulates with C3 (**Table 3.1**).

**Table 3.1** Comparison to other cervical vertebrae

| Vertebra | Similarities | Differences |
| --- | --- | --- |
| Atlas (C1) | | Posterior arch in place of lamina<br>Posterior tubercle in place of spinous process<br>Anterior arch with anterior process |
| Axis (C2) | Spinous process<br>Vertebral body | Articular processes in place of lamina<br>Dens/odontoid process |
| Both | Transverse processes with foramina for vertebral artery<br>Articular surfaces on lateral masses | No uncinate processes<br>Lateral masses in place of body |

# 3.2 Ligamentous Anatomy (Tables 3.2, 3.3; Figs. 3.4, 3.5)

# 3.3 Muscular Anatomy (Tables 3.4, 3.5; Figs. 3.6, 3.7)

# 3.4 Vascular Anatomy

**Table 3.2** Atlanto-occipital ligaments (**Figs. 3.5, 3.6**)

| Ligament | Origin | Insertion | Function |
|---|---|---|---|
| Anterior | | | |
| Anterior atlanto-occipital membrane (AAO) | Anterior aspect of atlas | Anterior rim of foramen magnum | Limits extension of head |
| Barkow's ligament | Anteromedial aspect of occipital condyle anterior to alar ligament | Anteromedial aspect of occipital condyle anterior to alar ligament | Limits extension of atlanto-occipital joint |
| Lateral atlanto-occipital ligament (LAO) | Anterolateral transverse process of axis | Jugular process of occipital bone | Limits lateral flexion of the head |
| Posterior | | | |
| Posterior atlanto-occipital membrane (PAO) | Posterior arch of atlas | Posterior rim of foramen magnum | Posterior reinforcement of joint |
| Tectorial membrane | Posterior axis | Upper surface of occipital bone anterior to foramen magnum | Restricts extension at atlanto-occipital joint (continuation of posterior longitudinal ligament) |
| Posterior atlanto-occipital membrane (PAO) | Posterior arch of atlas | Posterior rim of foramen magnum | Posterior reinforcement of joint |
| Nuchal ligament | Spinous process of C7 | Inferior projection of occipital bone | Restricts hyperflexion of cervical spine (continuation of supraspinous ligament) |

**Table 3.3** Atlantoaxial ligaments

| Ligament | Origin | Insertion | Function |
|---|---|---|---|
| Anterior | | | |
| Cruciate ligament (transverse atlantal ligament) | Lateral tubercle of atlas | Lateral tubercle of atlas of opposite site | Maintains stability of atlantoaxial junction by locking odontoid process against anterior arch of C1 Strongest ligament of the atlantoaxial joint |
| Alar ligaments | Lateral aspect of odontoid process | Base of skull | Limits hyperrotation and lateral bending on contralateral side |
| Transverse occipital ligament (TOL) | Inner aspect of occipital condyle | Inner aspect of occipital condyle | Sits posterosuperiorly to alar ligaments and assists them in support of craniocervical junction |
| Posterior | | | |
| Accessory atlantoaxial ligament | Medial dorsal surface of axis | Posterior to transverse ligament on lateral mass of atlas | Protection and support for branches of vertebral artery that supply the dens |
| Tectorial membrane | Posterior axis | Upper surface of occipital bone anterior to foramen magnum | Restricts flexion/extension at atlantoaxial joint |
| Nuchal ligament | Spinous process of C7 | Inferior projection of occipital bone | Restricts hyperflexion of cervical spine |

- Vertebral artery: arterial supply of C1 and C2:
  - Four segments (V1–V4).
  - Originates from subclavian artery:
    - Ascends between anterior scalene and longus colli muscles.
    - Reaches C6 vertebrae and enters transverse foramen.
  - Four segments (V1–V4): progresses superiorly:
    - V1: preforaminal:
      - Subclavian artery to transverse foramen of C6:
        - Despite a vertebral foramen in C7, the vertebral artery does not travel through it in a majority of individuals.
    - V2: foraminal:
      - Transverse foramen (C6) to C2 vertebrae.
  - Segments at the craniocervical junction:
    - V3: above C2:
      - C2 to dura mater.
    - V4: intradural:
      - Intradural to basilar artery (brainstem).

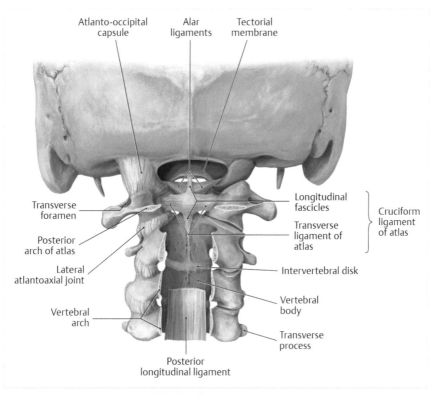

**Fig. 3.4** Internal ligaments of craniocervical junction. (Reproduced with permission from Baaj AA, Mummaneni PV, Uribe JS, Vaccaro AR, Greenberg MS, eds. Handbook of Spine Surgery. 2nd edition. New York, NY: Thieme; 2016)

- Feeding branches to C1 and C2:
  - Anterior spinal artery:
    - Single midline vessel.
    - Supplies anterior two-thirds of spinal cord within C1 and C2.
  - Posterior spinal artery:
    - Supplies posterior one-third of spinal cord within C1 and C2.
  - Anterior ascending artery:
    - Branch off vertebral arteries immediately caudal to axis.
    - Primary supply to odontoid.
    - Forms collateral system with posterior ascending artery.
  - Posterior ascending artery:
    - Branch off vertebral arteries caudal to axis.
    - Primary supply to odontoid.

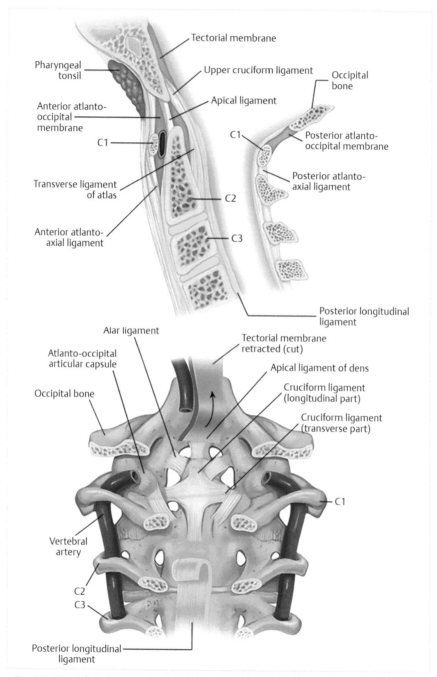

**Fig. 3.5** Sagittal view of external ligaments of craniocervical junction. (Reproduced with permission from An HS, Singh K, eds. Synopsis of Spine Surgery. 3rd ed. New York, NY: Thieme; 2016)

**Table 3.4** Suboccipital triangle (**Fig. 3.6**)

| Muscle | Origin | Insertion | Action | Innervation |
|---|---|---|---|---|
| Rectus capitis posterior (major) | Spine of C2 vertebrae (axis) | Inferior nuchal line | Extend, rotate, and laterally flex head | Suboccipital nerve (dorsal ramus of C1) |
| Rectus capitis posterior (minor) | Posterior tubercle of C1 vertebrae (C1) | Occipital bone | Extend and laterally flex head | Suboccipital nerve |
| Obliquus capitis | Transverse process of atlas | Occipital bone | Extend and laterally flex head | Suboccipital nerve |
| Obliquus capitis inferior | Spine of axis | Transverse process of atlas | Extend and laterally flex head | Suboccipital nerve |

**Table 3.5** Deep anterior neck muscles (**Fig. 3.7**)

| Muscle | Origin | Insertion | Action | Innervation |
|---|---|---|---|---|
| Longus capitis | Transverse process of C3–C6 | Basilar part of occipital bone | Flexion of neck at atlanto-occipital joint | C1–C4 nerve roots |
| Longus colli | Transverse process of C5–T3 | Anterior arch of atlas | Flexes head and neck | C2–C6 nerve roots |

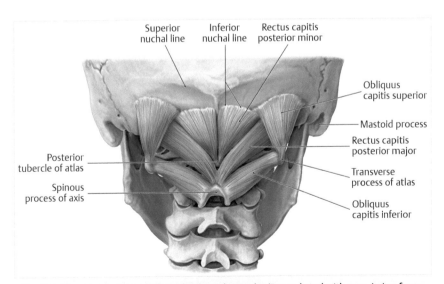

**Fig. 3.6** Muscular anatomy of the suboccipital triangle. (Reproduced with permission from Baaj AA, Mummaneni PV, Uribe JS, Vaccaro AR, Greenberg MS, eds. *Handbook of Spine Surgery*. 2nd ed. New York, NY: Thieme; 2016)

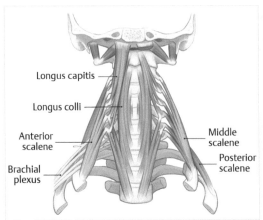

**Fig. 3.7** Deep anterior muscles of the neck.

Longus capitis

Longus colli

Anterior scalene

Middle scalene

Posterior scalene

Brachial plexus

- Posterior ascending arteries connect to form apical arcade at top of odontoid process.
- Forms collateral system with anterior ascending artery.
  ○ Anterior segmental medullary artery:
  - Small branches penetrating cervical vertebrae and spinal cord.
  ○ Posterior segmental medullary artery:
  - Small branches penetrating cervical vertebrae and spinal cord.

## 3.5  Neural Anatomy

- C1 and C2 nerve roots:
  - Exit above respective vertebrae.
  - Exhibit both ventral and dorsal rami:
    ○ Ventral rami: motor innervation for strap muscles.
    ○ Dorsal rami: motor innervation for suboccipital triangle muscles and sensation of the posterior scalp (**Fig. 3.8**).
- Cervical plexus:
  - Anterior rami of C1–C4.
  - Gives rise to ansa cervicalis.
    ○ Ventral rami of C1 form superior root:
    - Gives off branches to infrahyoid anterior neck muscles (strap muscles): omohyoid, sternohyoid, and sternothyroid.
    ○ Ventral rami of C2 join C3 to form inferior root:
    - Gives off branches to strap muscles: omohyoid, sternohyoid, and sternothyroid.

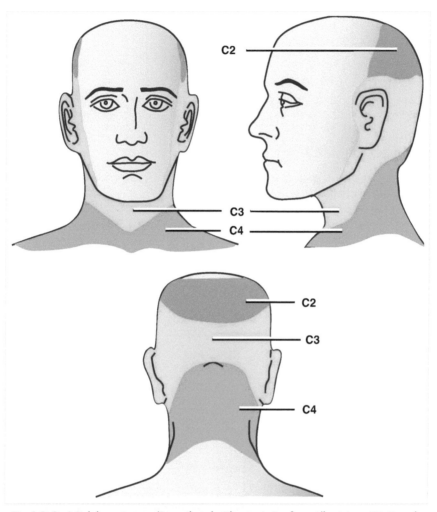

**Fig. 3.8** Occipital dermatomes. (Reproduced with permission from Albertstone CD, Benzel EC, Najm IM, Steinmetz M, eds. *Anatomic Basis of Neurologic Diagnosis.* New York, NY: Thieme; 2009)

## 3.6  Clinical and Surgical Pearls

- C1 and C2 nerve roots can be sacrificed with minimal consequences in occipital–cervical fusion and risk of occipital neuralgia.
- High-energy forces such as motor vehicle collisions can result in atlanto-occipital ligamentous injury:
  - Separates spinal column from occiput, frequently damaging the brainstem.

- Anomalous fusion of cervical vertebrae most commonly occurs between C1 and C2 or between C5 and C6.
- 3–15% of the population has an arcuate foramen:
  - Bony bridge covering the groove for vertebral artery (V3) entering C1:
    ◦ Caused by calcification of atlanto-occipital ligaments.
- C2 pedicles are narrow, increasing the risk for screw breach into the neural canal during occipitocervical fusion procedures.

## Suggested Readings

1.   An HS, Singh K. Synopsis of Spine Surgery. 3rd ed. New York, NY: Thieme; 2016
2.   Althoff B, Goldie IF. The arterial supply of the odontoid process of the axis. Acta Orthop Scand 1977;48(6):622–629
3.   Netter FH. Atlas of Human Anatomy. 6th ed. Philadelphia, PA: Saunders; 2014
4.   Tubbs RS, Hallock JD, Radcliff V, et al. Ligaments of the craniocervical junction. J Neurosurg Spine 2011;14(6):697–709

# 4 Cervical Spine Anatomy

*Fady Y. Hijji, Ankur S. Narain, Philip K. Louie, Daniel D. Bohl, and Kern Singh*

## 4.1 General Information

- C3–C7 are defined as the subaxial spine.
- Majority of flexion/extension of the neck and lateral bending occur here:
  - Maximal flexion occurs at C4/C5 and C5/C6.
  - Maximal lateral bending occurs at C2/C3, C3/C4, and C4/C5.
- Lordotic curvature: 16 to 25 degrees.
- Landmarks:
  - C2/C3: lower border of mandible.
  - C3: hyoid bone.
  - C4: thyroid cartilage.
  - C6: cricoid cartilage.

## 4.2 Bony Anatomy (Fig. 4.1)

- Vertebral body:
  - Concave superiorly.
  - Convex inferiorly.
- Uncinate process:
  - Directly interacts with adjacent vertebral body above.
  - Contain articular surfaces.
- Pedicle:
  - Angled medially and superiorly.
  - Pedicles smaller than those in thoracic and lumbar spine.
- Transverse process:
  - Contains transverse foramen:
    - **All** cervical vertebrae have transverse foramen.
    - Anterior to nerve root groove.
    - Allow for passage of vertebral artery.
  - C6 transverse process (Chassaignac's tubercle) is palpable.
- Lamina:
  - Bridge between lateral masses and spinous process.
- Lateral mass:
  - Lateral to junction between pedicle and lamina.
  - Contains the superior and inferior articular processes:

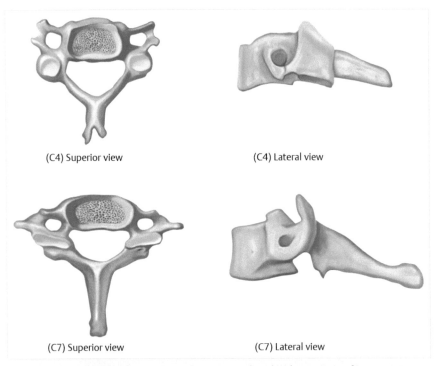

(C4) Superior view                    (C4) Lateral view

(C7) Superior view                    (C7) Lateral view

**Fig. 4.1** Bony anatomy of cervical vertebrae. (Reproduced with permission from An HS, Singh K, eds. Synopsis of Spine Surgery. 3rd ed. New York, NY: Thieme; 2016.)

- ◦ Creates the facet joint with the adjacent vertebral articular processes.
- ◦ Superior articular facets exhibit posteromedial orientation, transitioning to posterolateral with caudal progression:
  - • Supports more flexion/extension.
- Spinous process:
  - – Bifid from C3 to C5.
  - – C7 exhibits largest spinous process.

# 4.3 Ligamentous Anatomy

- Anterior ligamentous complex:
  - – Anterior longitudinal ligament (ALL):
    - ◦ Traverses along anterior surface of vertebral bodies.
    - ◦ Resists extension.
  - – Annulus fibrosis of the intervertebral disk.
- Middle ligamentous complex:
  - – Posterior longitudinal ligament (PLL):
    - ◦ Traverses along posterior surface of vertebral bodies.
    - ◦ Resists flexion.

- Annulus fibrosis.
- Posterior ligamentous complex:
  - Facet capsules:
    - Support facet joint for adjacent vertebra articulation and resist distractive forces.
  - Interspinous and supraspinous ligament:
    - Traverse between spinous processes:
      - Midline avascular plane.
    - Continuous with the ligamentous nuchae above C7.
  - Ligamentum flavum:
    - Deepest structure posteriorly prior to reaching spinal canal.
    - Connects the laminas of adjacent vertebrae.

## 4.4 Muscular Anatomy

- Fascial layers (**Fig. 4.2**):
  - Platysma:
    - Superficial muscle.
  - Superficial layer of deep cervical fascia:
    - Contains anterior neck muscles (except longus colli) and trapezius posteriorly.
  - Prevertebral layer of deep cervical fascia:
    - Contains all posterior neck muscles deep to trapezius.
    - Covers ALL and longus colli.
  - Pretracheal fascia:
    - Contains thyroid and trachea.
  - Carotid sheath:
    - Contains carotid artery, internal jugular vein, and vagus nerve (cranial nerve X).
- Muscular layers:
  - Anterior neck muscles (**Fig. 4.3; Tables 4.1 and 4.2**):
    - Divided into two regions: anterior neck and anterior cervical triangle:
      - Anterior cervical triangle primarily functions to move the hyoid bone.
  - Posterior neck muscles:
    - Divided into three regions: posterior neck, occipital triangle, and suboccipital triangle:
      - Posterior neck (**Table 4.3, Figs. 4.4, 4.5**).
      - Occipital triangle (**Table 4.4, Fig. 4.6**):
        - ❖ Borders: sternocleidomastoid (SCM; anterior), trapezius (posterior), and omohyoid (inferior).
      - Suboccipital triangle:
        - ❖ Borders: formed by the muscles it contains.
        - ❖ See Chapter 3.

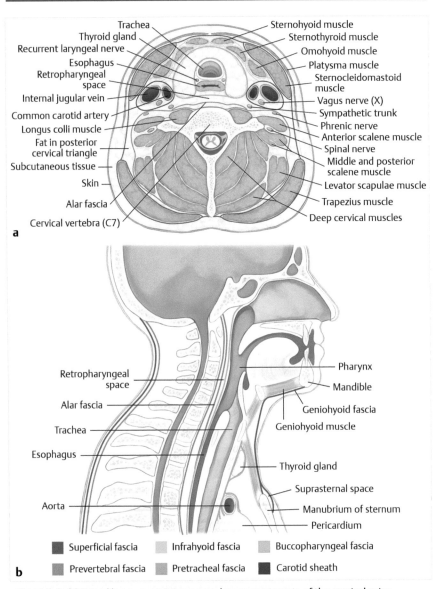

**Fig. 4.2 (a,b)** Fascial layers containing muscular compartments of the cervical spine.

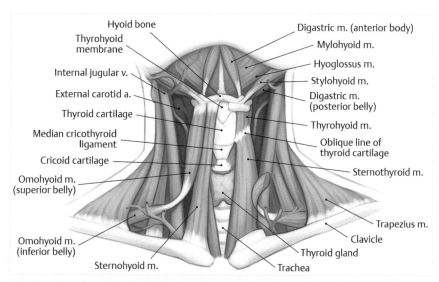

**Fig 4.3** Muscular anatomy of anterior neck.

**Table 4.1** Anterior neck

| Muscle | Origin | Insertion | Action | Innervation |
|---|---|---|---|---|
| Platysma | Deltoid and pectoralis major | Mandible | Lower jaw | Cranial nerve VII |
| Sternocleidomastoid (SCM) | Manubrium of sternum and clavicle | Mastoid process of skull | Turn head (left SCM turns head to the right) | Cranial nerve XI |

# 4.5  Vascular Anatomy

• Cervical region rich in vascular structures.
• Carotid sheath:
  – Within carotid triangle of anterior neck:
    ◦ Formed by SCM laterally, digastric superiorly, and omohyoid anteriorly.
  – Contains carotid artery (anteromedial), internal jugular vein (anterolateral), and vagus nerve (posterior between artery and vein).

**Table 4.2** Anterior cervical triangle

| Muscle | Origin | Insertion | Action | Innervation |
|---|---|---|---|---|
| Suprahyoid | | | | |
| Digastric | Mandible (anterior belly); mastoid notch of temporal bone (posterior belly) | Hyoid bone | Depresses mandible and elevates larynx | Cranial nerve V (anterior belly); cranial nerve VII (posterior belly) |
| Mylohyoid | Mandible | Hyoid bone | Depresses mandible, elevated hyoid | Cranial nerve V |
| Stylohyoid | Styloid process | Hyoid bone | Elevate hyoid | Cranial nerve VII |
| Geniohyoid | Mandible | Hyoid bone | Elevate hyoid | C1 |
| Infrahyoid (superficial) | | | | |
| Sternohyoid | Manubrium and clavicle | Hyoid bone | Depress hyoid | Ansa cervicalis (C1–C3) |
| Omohyoid | Suprascapular notch | Hyoid bone | Depress hyoid | Ansa cervicalis |
| Infrahyoid (deep) | | | | |
| Thyrohyoid | Thyroid cartilage | Hyoid bone | Depress hyoid | C1 |
| Sternothyroid | Manubrium of sternum | Hyoid bone | Depress hyoid and larynx | Ansa cervicalis |

**Table 4.3** Posterior neck

| Muscle | Origin | Insertion | Action | Innervation |
|---|---|---|---|---|
| Superficial (extrinsic) | | | | |
| Trapezius | Spinous processes of C7–T12 | Clavicle and scapula | Rotate and raise scapula | Cranial nerve XI |
| Superficial (intrinsic) | | | | |
| Splenius capitis | Ligamentum nuchae | Mastoid and nuchal line | Laterally flex and rotate neck | Dorsal rami of C4, C5, C6 |
| Deep (intrinsic) | | | | |
| Semispinalis capitis | Transverse process T1–T6 | Nuchal ridge | Extend head | Dorsal rami |

- Subclavian artery (**Fig. 4.7**):
  - Originates from aorta (left) or brachiocephalic trunk (right):
    - Traverses between anterior and middle scalene muscles.
  - Branches:
    - Vertebral artery:
      - Bilateral.
      - Primary arterial supply to cervical vertebrae and cord.

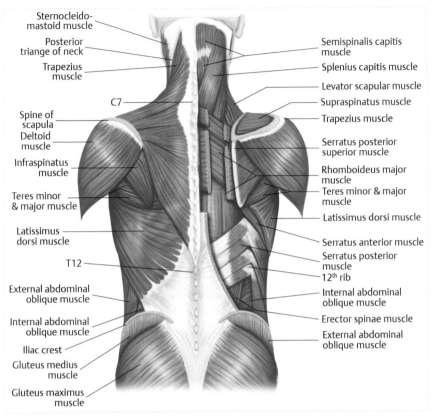

Sternocleido-
mastoid muscle

Posterior
triangle of neck

Trapezius
muscle

C7

Spine of
scapula

Deltoid
muscle

Infraspinatus
muscle

Teres minor
& major muscle

Latissimus
dorsi muscle

T12

External abdominal
oblique muscle

Internal abdominal
oblique muscle

Iliac crest

Gluteus medius
muscle

Gluteus maximus
muscle

Semispinalis capitis
muscle

Splenius capitis muscle

Levator scapular muscle

Supraspinatus muscle

Trapezius muscle

Serratus posterior
superior muscle

Rhomboideus major
muscle

Teres minor & major
muscle

Latissimus dorsi muscle

Serratus anterior muscle

Serratus posterior
muscle

12th rib

Internal abdominal
oblique muscle

Erector spinae muscle

External abdominal
oblique muscle

**Fig. 4.4** Muscular anatomy of superficial and deep posterior neck. (Reproduced with permission from An HS, Singh K, eds. Synopsis of Spine Surgery. 3rd ed. New York, NY: Thieme; 2016.)

- ○ Ascending cervical:
  - ▪ Travels with phrenic nerve.
  - ▪ Runs along anterior scalene muscle.
- ○ Superficial cervical:
  - ▪ Travels into posterior neck.
- ○ Deep cervical:
  - ▪ Anastomoses with occipital artery.
- • Vertebral artery (**Fig. 4.8**):
  - – Originates from subclavian artery:
    - ○ Ascends between anterior scalene and longus colli muscles.
    - ○ Reaches C6 vertebrae and enters transverse foramen.
  - – Four segments: progresses superiorly:

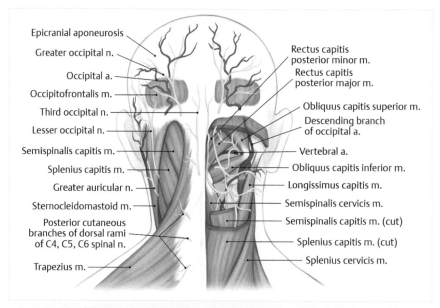

Epicranial aponeurosis
Greater occipital n.
Occipital a.
Occipitofrontalis m.
Third occipital n.
Lesser occipital n.
Semispinalis capitis m.
Splenius capitis m.
Greater auricular n.
Sternocleidomastoid m.
Posterior cutaneous branches of dorsal rami of C4, C5, C6 spinal n.
Trapezius m.

Rectus capitis posterior minor m.
Rectus capitis posterior major m.
Obliquus capitis superior m.
Descending branch of occipital a.
Vertebral a.
Obliquus capitis inferior m.
Longissimus capitis m.
Semispinalis cervicis m.
Semispinalis capitis m. (cut)
Splenius capitis m. (cut)
Splenius cervicis m.

**Fig. 4.5** Muscular anatomy of superficial and deep posterior neck and suboccipital triangle with associated nerves.

**Table 4.4** Occipital triangle

| Muscle | Origin | Insertion | Action | Innervation |
| --- | --- | --- | --- | --- |
| Anterior scalene | Transverse process of C3–C6 | First rib | Laterally flexes neck and raises first rib | C5–C8 nerve roots |
| Middle scalene | Transverse process of C2–C7 | First rib | Laterally flexes neck and raises First rib | C5–C8 nerve roots |
| Posterior scalene | Transverse process of C4–C6 | Second rib | Laterally flexes neck and raises second rib | C5–C8 nerve roots |

- V1: preforaminal:
  - Subclavian artery to transverse foramen (C6).
  - Despite a vertebral foramen in C7, the vertebral artery does not travel through it in a majority of individuals.
- V2: foraminal:
  - Transverse foramen (C6) to C2 vertebrae.
- V3: above C2:
  - C2 to dura mater.
- V4: intradural:
  - Intradural to basilar artery (brainstem).

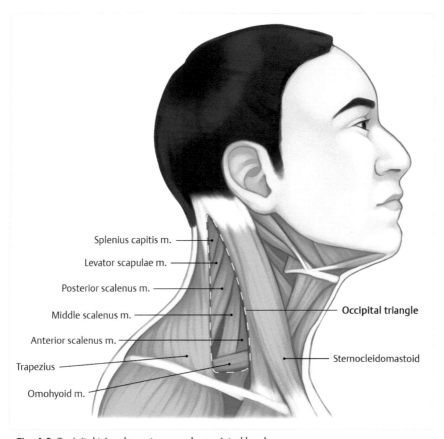

**Fig. 4.6** Occipital triangle anatomy and associated borders.

- Branches:
  - Anterior spinal artery.
  - Posterior spinal artery.
  - Anterior ascending artery:
    - Primary supply to odontoid.
  - Posterior ascending artery:
    - Primary supply to odontoid.
  - Anterior segmental medullary artery.
  - Posterior segmental medullary artery.
- Anterior spinal artery:
  - Originates from vertebral artery:
    - Branches at pontomedullary junction of brainstem.
    - Travels within ventral median fissure.

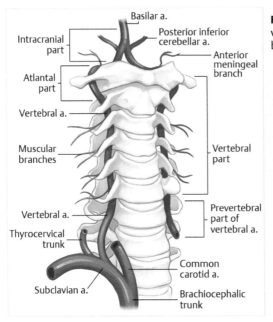

Basilar a.
Posterior inferior cerebellar a.
Intracranial part
Anterior meningeal branch
Atlantal part
Vertebral a.
Muscular branches
Vertebral part
Vertebral a.
Thyrocervical trunk
Prevertebral part of vertebral a.
Common carotid a.
Subclavian a.
Brachiocephalic trunk

**Fig. 4.7** Anatomy of the vertebral artery and associated branches.

- Single midline artery:
  - Feeds anterior two-thirds of spinal cord.
  - Communicates with branches of other arteries:
    - Anterior segmental medullary artery (from vertebral artery) at C3.
    - Anterior cervical artery (from inferior thyroid artery) at C6.
- Posterior spinal artery:
  - Originates from vertebral artery:
    - Branches at medulla.
  - Bilateral artery:
    - Feeds posterior one-third of spinal cord.
    - Travels within posterolateral sulci of spinal cord.

## 4.6 Neural Anatomy

- Cervical spinal cord decreases in diameter cranially.
- Nerve roots:
  - Exit anterolateral to superior facet.
  - C3–C7 nerve roots exit **above** the pedicle of their respective vertebrae.
  - C8 exits **below** C7 vertebra (above T1 pedicle).
  - Dorsal (posterior) rami provide sensation for majority of posterior neck and head.
  - Ventral (anterior) rami form two nerve plexuses:
    - Cervical plexus.
    - Brachial plexus.

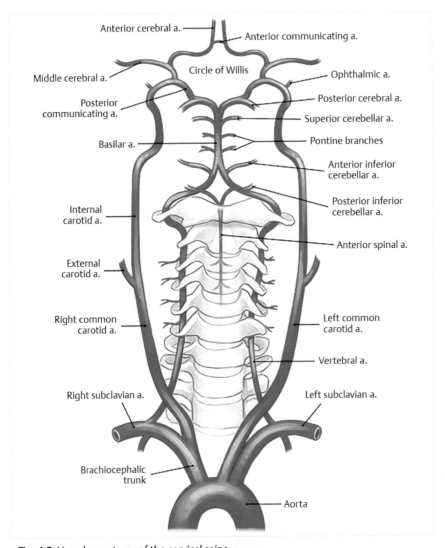

**Fig. 4.8** Vascular anatomy of the cervical spine.

- Cervical plexus (**Fig. 4.9**):
  - Anterior rami of C1–C4.
  - Gives rise to:
    - Ansa cervicalis:
      - Described in Chapter 3.
    - Phrenic nerve (C3–C5):
      - Innervates diaphragm.
    - Cutaneous nerves of posterior head and neck.

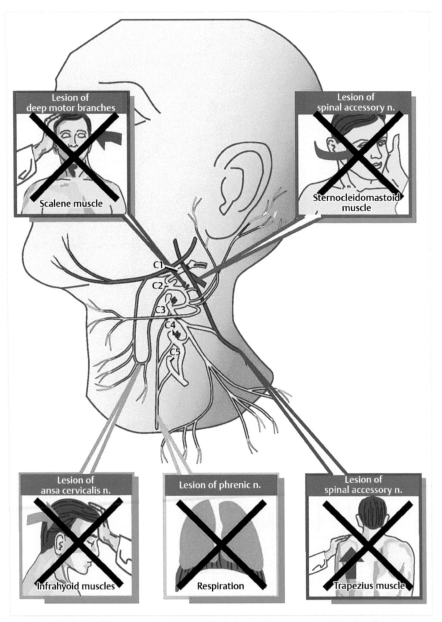

**Fig. 4.9** Cervical plexus with corresponding nerve roots and terminal innervations. (Reproduced with permission from Albertstone CD, Benzel EC, Najm IM, Steinmetz M, eds. Anatomic Basis of Neurologic Diagnosis. New York, NY: Thieme; 2009.)

- Brachial plexus (**Fig. 4.10**):
  - Anterior rami of C5–T1 (**Tables 4.5, 4.6**).
  - Divided into five segments:
    - Roots.
    - Trunks.
    - Divisions.
    - Cords.
    - Terminal nerves.

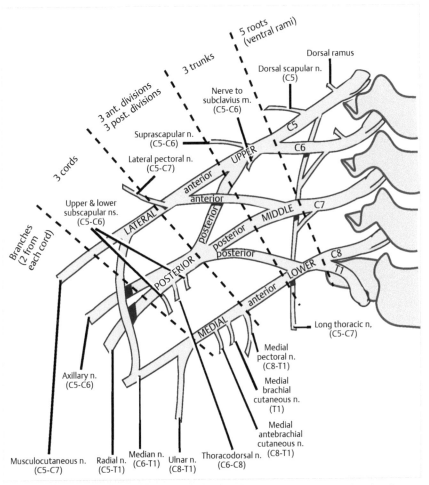

**Fig. 4.10** Brachial plexus divided by segments and branching nerves. (Reproduced with permission from Albertstone CD, Benzel EC, Najm IM, Steinmetz M, eds. Anatomic Basis of Neurologic Diagnosis. New York, NY: Thieme; 2009.)

- Cervical dermatomes:
  - Each nerve root provides the predominant sensory innervation for a specific area of skin.
  - Important dermatomes:
    - C5: lateral shoulder and arm.
    - C6: lateral forearm and thumb.
    - C7: index and middle fingers.
    - C8: ring and little fingers.
    - T1: medial forearm.

**Table 4.5** Brachial plexus

| Level | Nerve | Origin | Motor | Sensory |
|---|---|---|---|---|
| Roots | Long thoracic nerve | C5, C6, C7 | Serratus anterior | None |
| | Dorsal scapular nerve | C4, C5 | Levator scapulae, rhomboids | None |
| | Phrenic nerve (contribution) | C5 | Diaphragm | Diaphragm |
| Trunks | Suprascapular nerve | C5, C6 | Supraspinatus and infraspinatus | None |
| | Nerve to subclavius | C5, C6 | Subclavius | |
| Cords | Lateral pectoral nerve | C5, C6, C7 | Pectoralis major and minor | None |
| | Thoracodorsal nerve | C6, C7, C8 | Latissimus dorsi | None |
| | Inferior subscapular nerve | C5, C6 | Subscapularis and teres major | None |
| | Superior subscapular nerve | C5, C6 | Subscapularis | None |
| | Medial pectoral nerve | C8, T1 | Pectoralis major and minor | None |
| | Medial cutaneous nerve of arm | C8, T1 | None | Medial aspect of upper arm overlying biceps brachii |
| | Medial cutaneous nerve of forearm | C8, T1 | | Ulnar aspect of volar forearm |

(Continued)

**Table 4.5** (Continued)

| Level | Nerve | Origin | Motor | Sensory |
|---|---|---|---|---|
| Terminal branches | Axillary nerve | C5, C6 | Deltoid and teres minor | Deltoid and superior posterior arm |
| | Musculocutaneous nerve | C5, C6, C7 | Anterior compartment of upper arm (biceps brachii, brachialis) | Lateral forearm (lateral antebrachial cutaneous nerve branch) |
| | Median nerve | C5–T1 | Anterior compartment of forearm, except flexor carpi ulnaris and ulnar side of flexor digitorum profundus | Volar aspect of first three digits, lateral two-thirds of palm |
| | Radial nerve | C5–T1 | Posterior compartment of arm and forearm | Posterior arm and forearm, dorsal aspect of first three digits, lateral two-thirds of dorsum of hand |
| | Ulnar nerve | C8, T1 | Most intrinsic muscles of the hand, flexor carpi ulnaris, ulnar side of flexor digitorum profundus | Medial side of hand and fourth and fifth digits |

# 4.7 Clinical and Surgical Pearls

• Cervical disk herniation most commonly occurs at C5–C6 and C6–C7.
• Due to smaller pedicles in the cervical spine, screw placement here is not feasible:
  - Magerl's technique used for screw placement in cervical lateral masses:
    ○ Vertebral artery at risk; to avoid risk, drill is positioned slightly medial to midpoint of lateral mass, and angled superiorly and laterally.

**Table 4.6** Common brachial plexus injuries

| Disorder | Etiology | Nerves | Physical examination |
|---|---|---|---|
| Winged scapula | Avulsion of proximal C5, C6 nerve roots | • Long thoracic nerve loss<br>• Dorsal scapular nerve loss<br>• Phrenic nerve deficiency (loss of serratus anterior and rhomboids) | Medial displacement of scapula, flail arm, elevated hemidiaphragm |
| Erb's palsy | Traction or avulsion of upper trunk (C5, C6) | • Axillary nerve deficiency (weak deltoid/teres minor)<br>• Suprascapular nerve deficiency (weak infra/supraspinatus)<br>• Musculocutaneous nerve deficiency (weak biceps)<br>• Radial nerve deficiency (weak brachioradialis, supinator) | Arm internally rotated, adducted, pronated, and extended at elbow |
| Klumpke's palsy | Traction or avulsion of lower trunk (C8, T1) | • Ulnar nerve deficiency (loss of hand intrinsics)<br>• Median nerve deficiency (loss of wrist flexors) | Wrist extended, metacarpophalangeal (MCP) joints extended, flexion of proximal interphalangeal (PIP) joints |
| Claw hand | Damage to peripheral ulnar nerve | • Ulnar nerve deficiency (loss of hand intrinsics) | Fourth and fifth digits extended at MCP and flexed at PIP |

# 5 Thoracic Spine

*Catherine Maloney, Fady Y. Hijji, Ankur S. Narain, Philip K. Louie, Daniel D. Bohl, and Kern Singh*

## 5.1 General Information

- T1–T12 are defined as the thoracic vertebrae (**Table 5.1**):
- Kyphotic curvature: 20–40 degrees:
  - Apex of kyphosis at T7–T8:
    - Pathologic kyphosis can have an apex at any level.
- Articulate with their corresponding ribs at facet joints, limited range of motion:
  - Flexion–extension minimal at T1–T2; maximum T12–L1.
  - Axial rotation minimal at thoracolumbar junction; maximum at T12.
- Wedge shaped with anterior height shorter than posterior height.
- Width of vertebral canal is smallest in the thoracic vertebrae.

## 5.2 Bony Anatomy (Fig. 5.1)

- Vertebral body:
  - Anterior border of intervertebral foramen.
  - Forms articulation with ribs:
    - Each rib articulates with two vertebral bodies:
      - Inferior costal demifacet of superior vertebral body and superior costal facet of inferior vertebral body.

**Table 5.1** Thoracic landmarks

| Vertebrae | Associated structure |
|---|---|
| T1 | Sternoclavicular joint |
| T1–T2 | Superior angle of the scapula |
| T2 | Jugular notch |
| T3 | Base of the spine of the scapula |
| T4 | Sternal angle of Louis |
| T5–T9 | Body of the sternum |
| T7 | Inferior angle of the scapula |
| T8 | Level at which the inferior vena cava passes through the diaphragm |
| T9 | Xiphisternal junction |
| T9–L3 | Costal margin |
| T10 | Esophagus passes through diaphragm |
| T12 | Aorta, thoracic duct, and azygous vein pass through diaphragm |

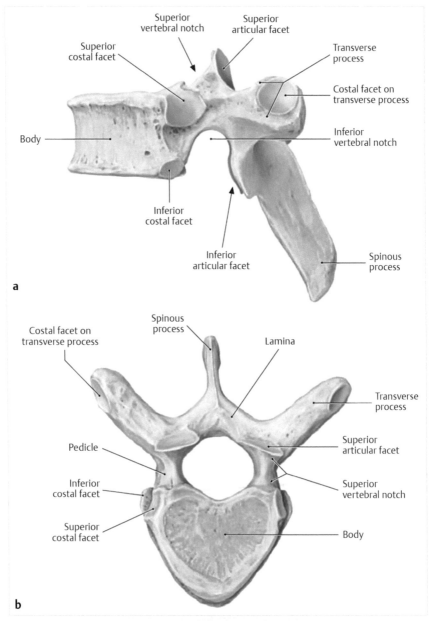

**Fig. 5.1** Lateral **(a)** and superior **(b)** views of the thoracic vertebrae. (Reproduced with permission from Baaj AA, Mummaneni PV, Uribe JS, Vaccaro AR, Greenberg MS, eds. Handbook of Spine Surgery. 2nd ed. New York, NY: Thieme; 2016.)

– Superior costal demifacet:
  ○ Superoposterior edge of vertebral body.
  ○ Articulates with corresponding rib of same number.
  ○ Exceptions:
    ▪ Superior costal facet of T1 is not a demifacet:
      ❖ First rib only articulates with T1.
    ▪ T10 has one pair of complete costal facets located between the vertebral body and pedicle.
    ▪ T11 and T12 have one pair of complete costal facets located on the pedicles.
  – Inferior costal demifacet:
    ○ Inferoposterior edge of vertebral body.
    ○ Articulates with head of rib below.
• Pedicle:
  – Height of pedicle is double that of the width.
  – Inferior notch is superior border of intervertebral foramen.
  – Superior notch is inferior border of intervertebral foramen.
  – Pedicle diameter is maximal at T1 and minimal at T6:
    ○ Diameter gradually increases again from T6.
• Superior articular process:
  – Faces posterolaterally.
  – Articulates with inferior articular process of adjacent superior vertebrae.
• Inferior articular process:
  – Faces anteromedially.
  – Articulates with superior articular process of adjacent inferior vertebrae.
• Lamina.
• Posterior border of vertebral foramen.
• Transverse process:
  – Forms the costotransverse joint.
  – T1–T10 have a costal facet on transverse process that articulates with tubercle of rib.
• Spinous process:
  – Long, points downward.
  – Becomes level with body of vertebrae below.

## 5.3 Ligamentous Anatomy

• Radiate ligament of head of rib:
  – Attaches head of rib to bodies and disk.
  – Reinforces costovertebral joint anteriorly.

- Costotransverse ligament:
  - Attaches neck of rib to transverse process.
- Superior costotransverse ligament:
  - Attaches rib to transverse process of superior vertebrae.
- Intratransverse ligament:
  - Fibrous cords that join adjacent thoracic vertebrae and blend with adjacent back muscles.
- Lateral costotransverse ligament:
  - Attaches transverse process to tubercle of rib.

# 5.4 Muscular Anatomy (Tables 5.2–5.4) Vascular Anatomy (Fig. 5.2)

- Less blood supply to thoracic spinal cord than cervical and lumbar regions:
  - Watershed region in midthoracic spinal cord:
    - Poorly vascularized area.
    - Between T4 and T9, least profuse blood supply; narrowest region of spinal canal.

**Table 5.2** Superficial layers of the back

| Muscle | Origin | Insertion | Action | Innervation |
|---|---|---|---|---|
| Trapezius (upper, middle, and lower divisions) | Upper division: medial one-third of superior nuchal line, external occipital protuberance, ligamentum nuchae, spinous processes of C7 Middle division: spinous process of T1–T5 Lower division: spinous process of T6–T12 | Upper division: lateral one-third of clavicle and acromion process of scapula Middle division: superior border of spine of scapula Lower division: medial one-third of spine of scapula | Upper division: upward rotation of scapula and elevation of scapula Middle division: retraction of scapula Lower division: upward rotation of scapula and depression of scapula | Cranial nerve XI C3–C4 dorsal rami (for proprioception) |
| Latissimus dorsi | Spinous processes of T7–L5, lower three or four ribs, posterior one-third of iliac crest | Floor of intertubercular groove | Extension and internal (medial) rotation of arm | Thoracodorsal nerve (C7–C8) |
| Rhomboid major | Spinous processes of T2–T5 | Medial border of scapula (inferior to spine of scapula) | Retraction, elevation, and rotation of scapula | Dorsal scapular nerve (C5) |
| Rhomboid minor | Inferior end of ligamentum nuchae, spinous processes of C7–T1 | Medial border of scapula | Retraction, elevation, and rotation of scapula | Dorsal scapular nerve (C5) |

**Table 5.3** Intermediate layers of the back

| Muscle | Origin | Insertion | Action | Innervation |
|---|---|---|---|---|
| Serratus posterior superior | Ligamentum nuchae, spinous processes of C7–T3 | Ribs 2–5 (lateral to angle of rib) | Elevation of upper ribs | T1–T4 ventral rami |
| Serratus posteroinferior | Thoracolumbar fascia, spinous processes of T11–L2 | Ribs 9–12 (lateral to the angle of rib) | Depression of lower ribs | T9–T12 ventral rami |
| Iliocostalis thoracis (erector spinae) | Superior borders of the angles of the lower six ribs | Angles of upper six or seven ribs and transverse process of C7 | Extension and lateral flexion of trunk and neck | C4–S5 dorsal rami |
| Longissimus thoracis (erector spinae) | Transverse process and spinous process of lumbar vertebrae, sacrum, and iliac crest | Transverse process of T1–T12 | Extension and lateral flexion of trunk and neck | C1–S1 dorsal rami |
| Spinalis thoracis (erector spinae) | Spinous process of T11–L3 | Spinous processes of T3–T8 | Extension and lateral flexion of trunk and neck | C2–L3 dorsal rami |

**Table 5.4** Deep layers of the back

| Muscle | Origin | Insertion | Action | Innervation |
|---|---|---|---|---|
| Semispinalis thoracis | Transverse processes of C7–T12 | Semispinalis capitis: back of skull between nuchal lines; semispinalis cervicis and thoracis: spinous processes of four to six vertebrae above origin | Extension lateral flexion, and contralateral rotation of trunk | C1–T12 dorsal rami |
| Thoracic interspinales | Spinous processes of thoracic vertebrae | Adjacent spinous process | Extension of spine | Dorsal rami of spinal nerves of region |
| Thoracic intertransversarii | Transverse process of vertebrae | Adjacent transverse process | Assist with lateral flexion of spine | Dorsal rami of spinal nerves of region |
| Multifidus | Sacrum, ilium, transverse processes of T1–T12, and articular processes of C4–C7 | Spinous processes of superior vertebrae, spanning two to four segments | Stabilize vertebral column | Dorsal rami of spinal nerves of region |

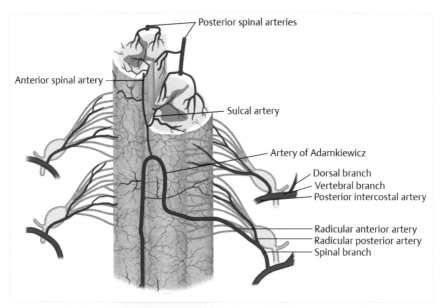

**Fig. 5.2** Vascularization of the spinal cord. Note the origin of the artery of Adamkiewicz from the left posterior intercostal artery.

- Anterior spinal artery:
  - Supplies ventral two-thirds of thoracic cord.
  - Originates from vertebral artery in region of medulla oblongata.
- Anterior medial spinal artery:
  - Continuation of the anterior spinal artery below T4.
- Posterolateral spinal arteries:
  - Originate from vertebral arteries.
  - Descend toward lower cervical and upper thoracic region.
- Posterior spinal arteries:
  - Paired arteries originating from vertebral arteries that branch at various levels to form the posterolateral arterial plexus.
  - Supply posterior one-third of cord (dorsal white columns and posterior portion of dorsal gray columns).
- Radicular arteries:
  - Originate from intercostal arteries at level of costotransverse joint:
    ◦ Intercostal arteries arise from the subclavian artery and thoracic aorta.
  - Enter vertebral canal through intervertebral foramina:
    ◦ Form anterior and posterior radicular arteries:
      ▪ Supply anterior and posterior spinal arteries.
- Radicular artery of Adamkiewicz:

- Largest segmental artery:
  - Typically arises from a left posterior intercostal artery.
  - Enters the spinal canal between T9 and T12.
- Major blood supply to inferior two-thirds of spinal cord.
- Usually travels with ventral roots of T9, T10, or T11.

## 5.5  Neural Anatomy

- Spinal cord enlarges between T9 and T12 (lumbar enlargement).
- Thoracic spinal nerves:
  - Exit **below** the pedicle of the corresponding numbered vertebrae.
  - Form from dorsal and ventral roots in the intervertebral foramen region.
  - Spinal nerve divides in the foramen into dorsal and ventral rami:
    - Ventral rami continue as intercostal nerves:
      - Innervate intermediate back muscle layers.
    - Dorsal rami provide cutaneous sensation and innervation of deep back muscles and thoracic facet joints.
- Thoracic neurovascular bundle:
  - Contains a posterior intercostal vein, posterior intercostal artery, and ventral rami of a spinal nerve.
  - Lies inferior to each rib.
  - Vein, artery, nerve (V-A-N) relationship from superior to inferior.
- Thoracic sinuvertebral nerves:
  - Three branches.
    - Ascending.
    - Descending.
    - Transverse.
  - Recurrent branches of ventral rami.
  - Mixed nerves; provide pain sensation to ventral surface of dura mater, intervertebral disk, posterior longitudinal ligaments, and intervertebral disk.
- Sympathetic trunk (**Fig. 5.3**):
  - Thoracic sympathetic trunk is located along anterior surface of rib head.
  - Each ganglia (T1–L2) in chain gives off a ramus communicans:
    - Ramus communicans merges with spinal nerve distal to where the anterior and posterior roots join.
- Thoracic dermatomes:
  - Lateral and anterior cutaneous branches of the intercostal nerves innervate skin of thorax.
  - Important dermatomes:
    - T4 dermatome: nipple (*note*: nipple may sit lower in females).
    - T6 dermatome: xiphoid process.
    - T10 dermatome: umbilicus.

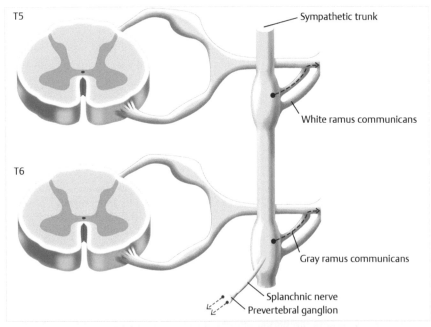

**Fig. 5.3** Thoracic vertebrae and the sympathetic trunk. Note the merging of the sympathetic root distal to the merging of the anterior and posterior roots.

# 5.6 Clinical and Surgical Pearls

- Ending spinal instrumentation at the thoracic kyphotic apex can lead to early instrumentation failure.
- Fractures above midthoracic region are not common: suspect osteolytic tumor rather than benign fracture.
- Collateral blood flow to the thoracic cord comes from the internal and lateral thoracic arteries:
  - Prevents infarction if blood supply from the aorta is interrupted.

## Suggested Readings

1. Yoganandan N, Halliday AL, Dickman CA, Benzel E. Practical anatomy and fundamental biomechanics. In: Benzel EC, ed. Spine Surgery Techniques, Complication Avoidance, and Management. 2nd ed. Philadelphia, PA: Elsevier; 2005:109–135
2. Netter FH. Atlas of Human Anatomy. 6th ed. Philadelphia, PA: Saunders; 2014
3. An HS, Singh K. Synopsis of Spine Surgery. 3rd ed. New York, NY: Thieme; 2016

# 6 Lumbar Spine Anatomy

*Melissa G. Goczalk, Ankur S. Narain, Fady Y. Hijji, Philip K. Louie, Daniel D. Bohl, and Kern Singh*

## 6.1 General Information

• Anatomy and function:
  - Lordotic curvature.
  - Long transverse processes for muscle attachment.
  - Lacks facets for rib articulation.
  - Supports weight of trunk.
  - Allow flexion, extension, lateral flexion, and rotation of spine.
• Landmarks:
  - L1: conus medullaris.
  - L3: umbilicus.
  - L4: iliac crests, aortic bifurcation.

## 6.2 Bony Anatomy (Fig. 6.1)

• Vertebral body:
  - Cylindrically shaped and widest transversely.
• Vertebral foramen:
  - Triangular spinal canal.
• Pedicles:
  - Connect vertebral body to lamina.
  - Directed posteriorly and located in the middle one-third of the transverse process.
• Transverse processes:
  - Thin and long from L1 to L4.
  - Large and cone-shaped at L5 due to iliolumbar ligament attachment to pelvic bones.
• Facet joints:
  - L1–L4 facets are sagittally oriented to limit axial rotation.
  - L5 facet is more coronal and resists anteroposterior movement.
  - Prominent pars interarticularis.
• Lamina:
  - Connect spinous process to pedicles.
• Spinous process:
  - Broad and thick orientation.

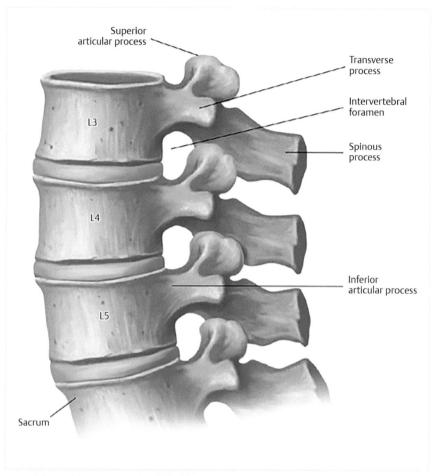

**Fig. 6.1** Bony anatomy of the lumbar vertebrae.

# 6.3 Ligamentous Anatomy (Fig. 6.2)

- Anterior longitudinal ligament:
  - Located on the anterior surface of vertebral bodies.
  - Functions include limiting spine extension and securing intervertebral disks.
- Posterior longitudinal ligament:
  - Located on the posterior surface of vertebral bodies.
  - Limits spine flexion and secures intervertebral disks.

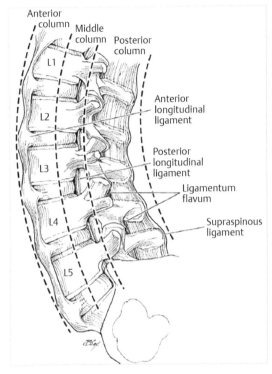

**Fig. 6.2** Ligamentous anatomy of the lumbar spine. (Reproduced with permission from Baaj AA, Mummaneni PV, Uribe JS, Vaccaro AR, Greenberg MS, eds. Handbook of Spine Surgery. 2nd ed. New York, NY: Thieme; 2016.)

- Ligamentum flavum:
  - Spans posterior aspect of the inferior lamina to the anterior aspect of the superior lamina.
  - Limits laminar flexion and separation.
- Supraspinous ligament:
  - Spans the tips of spinous processes; terminates at L3.
- Interspinous ligament:
  - Connect adjacent spinous processes; oriented obliquely.

# 6.4 Muscular Anatomy (Tables 6.1–6.6, Figs. 6.3–6.5)

# 6.5 Vascular Anatomy (Table 6.7)

# 6.6 Neural Anatomy (Tables 6.8 and 6.9, Figs. 6.6, 6.7)

- Five pairs of lumbar spinal nerves:
  - Exit below corresponding vertebral level.

**Table 6.1** Superficial extrinsic back muscles

| Muscle | Origin | Insertion | Action | Innervation |
| --- | --- | --- | --- | --- |
| Trapezius | Spinous processes of C7–T12 | Clavicle, scapula | Rotate scapula | Cranial nerve XI |
| Latissimus dorsi | Spinous processes of T6–T12, lumbar spine, sacrum, iliac crests, ribs 9–12 | Intertubercular sulcus of humerus | Extend, adduct, and medically rotate humerus | Thoracodorsal nerve |
| Levator scapulae | Transverse processes of C1–C4 | Medial scapulae | Elevate scapula | Dorsal scapular nerve |
| Rhomboid minor | Spinous processes of C7–T1 | Scapular spine | Adduct scapula | Dorsal scapular nerve |
| Rhomboid major | Spinous processes of T2–T5 | Medial border of scapula | Adduct scapula | Dorsal scapular nerve |
| Serratus posterosuperior | Spinous processes of C7–T5 | Upper border of ribs 2–5 | Elevate ribs | Intercostal nerves T1–T4 |
| Serratus posterior inferior | Spinous processes of T11–L3 | Lower border of ribs 9–12 | Depress ribs | Intercostal nerves T9–T12 |

**Table 6.2** Deep intrinsic back muscles: spinotransverse group

| Muscle | Origin | Insertion | Action | Innervation |
| --- | --- | --- | --- | --- |
| Splenius capitis | Ligamentum nuchae | Mastoid and nuchal line | Laterally flex and rotate ipsilateral neck | Dorsal rami of inferior cervical nerves |
| Splenius cervicis | Spinous processes of T1–T6 | Transverse processes of C1–C4 | Laterally flex and rotate ipsilateral neck | Dorsal rami of inferior cervical nerves |

**Table 6.3** Deep intrinsic back muscles: sacrospinalis group

| Muscle | Origin | Insertion | Action | Innervation |
| --- | --- | --- | --- | --- |
| Iliocostalis lumborum | Sacrum, spinous processes of lumbar and lower thoracic vertebrae, supraspinous ligaments, and iliac crests | Lower six to seven ribs | Bilateral: vertebral column and head extension Unilateral: vertebral column lateral flexion | Dorsal primary rami |
| Longissimus thoracis | Transverse processes of lumbar vertebrae | Transverse processes of thoracic vertebrae | Bilateral: vertebral column and head extension Unilateral: vertebral column lateral flexion | Dorsal primary rami |
| Spinalis thoracis | Spinous processes of T10–L2 | Spinous processes of T1–T8 | Bilateral: vertebral column and head extension Unilateral: vertebral column lateral flexion | Dorsal primary rami |

**Table 6.4**  Deep intrinsic back muscles: transversospinales group

| Muscle | Origin | Insertion | Action | Innervation |
|---|---|---|---|---|
| Semispinalis cervicis | Transverse processes | Spinous processes | Extend, rotate contralateral side | Dorsal primary rami |
| Semispinalis thoracic | Transverse processes | Spinous processes | Extend, rotate contralateral side | Dorsal primary rami |
| Semispinalis capitis | Transverse processes of T1–T6 | Nuchal ridge | Extend, rotate contralateral side | Dorsal primary rami |
| Multifidus | Transverse processes of C2–S4 | Spinous processes | Contralateral lateral flexion and rotation | Dorsal primary rami |
| Rotatores | Transverse processes | Spinous processes of superior vertebral level | Rotate contralateral superior vertebrae | Dorsal primary rami |
| Interspinales | Spinous processes | Spinous processes of superior vertebral level | Extend vertebral column | Dorsal primary rami |
| Intertrans-versarii | Transverse processes | Transverse processes of superior vertebral level | Lateral flex vertebral column | Dorsal primary rami |

**Table 6.5**  Anterolateral abdominal wall

| Muscle | Origin | Insertion | Action | Innervation |
|---|---|---|---|---|
| Rectus abdominis | Pubic crest, pubic tubercle, pubic symphysis | Costal cartilages of ribs 5–7 and xiphoid process | Compress abdominal contents, flex vertebral column, tense abdominal wall | Anterior rami of T7–T12 |
| External oblique | Anterior angles of ribs 5–12 | Iliac crest and aponeurosis to linea alba | Compress abdominal contents, flex trunk | Anterior rami of T7–T12 |
| Internal oblique | Thoracolumbar fascia, iliac crests, inguinal ligament | Inferior border of lower ribs, aponeurosis to linea alba, pubic crest, pectineal line | Compress abdominal contents, flex trunk | Anterior rami of T7–T12 and L1 |
| Transversus abdominis | Thoracolumbar fascia, iliac crests, inguinal ligament, costal cartilages of ribs 7–12 | Aponeurosis to linea alba, pubic crest, pectineal line | Compress abdominal contents | Anterior rami of T7–T12 and L1 |

**Table 6.6** Posterior abdominal wall muscles

| Muscle | Origin | Insertion | Action | Innervation |
|--------|--------|-----------|--------|-------------|
| Iliacus | Iliac fossa, anterior sacroiliac and iliolumbar ligaments, and sacrum | Lesser trochanter of femur | Flexion of thigh at hip | Femoral nerve |
| Psoas major | Vertebral bodies of T12 and L1–L5, transverse processes of lumbar vertebrae, and intervertebral disks of T12 and L1–L5 | Lesser trochanter of femur | Flexion of thigh at hip | Anterior rami of L1–L3 |
| Psoas minor | Vertebral bodies and intervertebral disks of T12 and L1 | Pectineal line of pelvic brim and iliopubic eminence | Flexion of lumbar vertebral column | Anterior rami of L1 |
| Quadratus lumborum | Transverse process of L5, iliolumbar ligament, iliac crest | Transverse process of L1–L4 and inferior border of rib 12 | Depress and stabilize rib 12 and lateral bending of trunk | Anterior rami of T12 and L1–L4 |

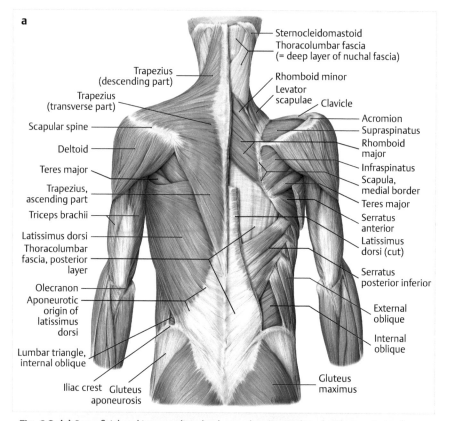

**Fig. 6.3 (a)** Superficial and intermediate back muscles. (Reproduced with permission from Gilroy A, MacPherson B, Schünke M et al., eds. Atlas of Anatomy. 3rd Edition. New York, NY: Thieme; 2017.)

(Continued)

**b**

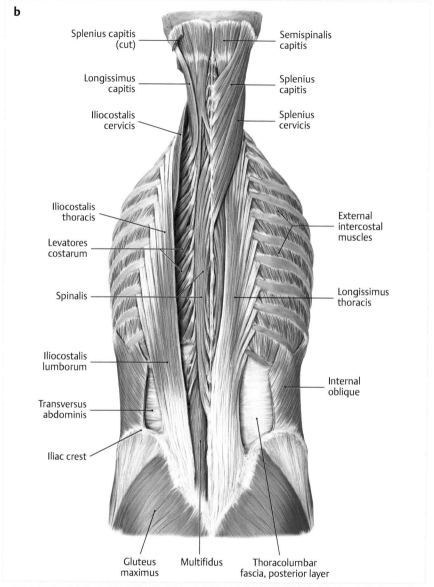

**Fig. 6.3** (*Continued*) **(b)** Intermediate and deep back muscles. (Reproduced with permission from Gilroy A, MacPherson B, Schünke M et al., eds. Atlas of Anatomy. 3rd Edition. New York, NY: Thieme; 2017.)

(*Continued*)

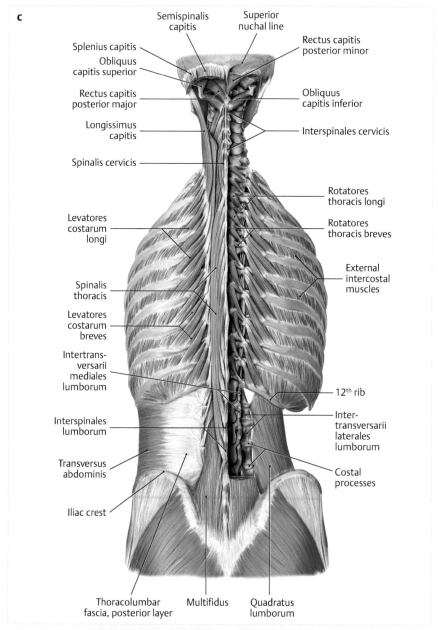

**Fig. 6.3** (*Continued*) **(c)** Deep back muscles. (Reproduced with permission from Gilroy A, MacPherson B, Schünke M et al., eds. Atlas of Anatomy. 3rd Edition. New York, NY: Thieme; 2017.)

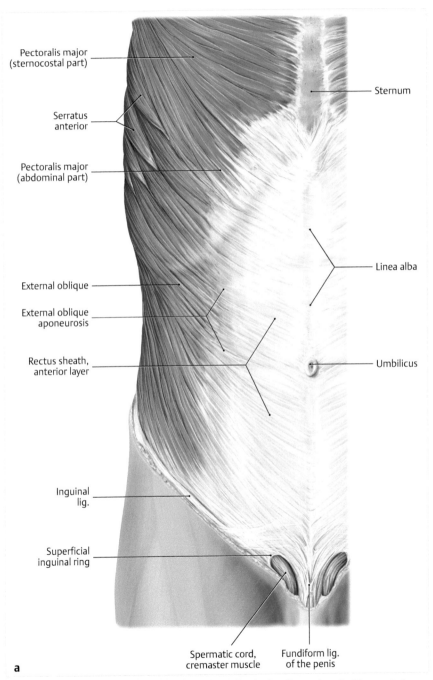

Pectoralis major
(sternocostal part)

Sternum

Serratus
anterior

Pectoralis major
(abdominal part)

Linea alba

External oblique

External oblique
aponeurosis

Rectus sheath,
anterior layer

Umbilicus

Inguinal
lig.

Superficial
inguinal ring

Spermatic cord,
cremaster muscle

Fundiform lig.
of the penis

a

**Fig. 6.4 (a)** Superficial anterolateral abdominal wall muscles. (Reproduced with permission from Gilroy A, MacPherson B, Schünke M et al., ed. Atlas of Anatomy. 3rd Edition. New York, NY: Thieme; 2017.)

*(Continued)*

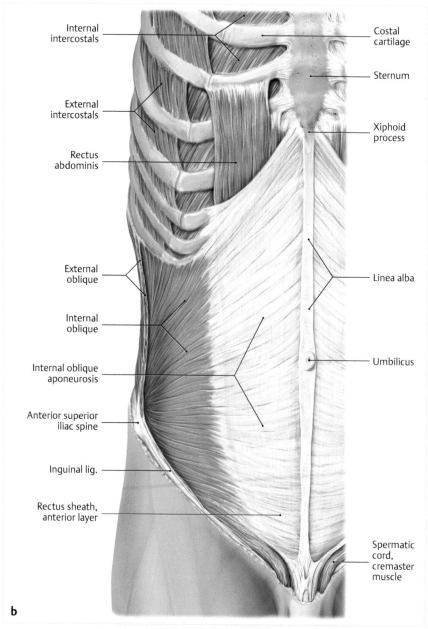

b

**Fig. 6.4** (*Continued*) **(b)** Intermediate anterolateral abdominal wall muscles. (Reproduced with permission from Gilroy A, MacPherson B, Schünke M et al., ed. Atlas of Anatomy. 3rd Edition. New York, NY: Thieme; 2017.)

(*Continued*)

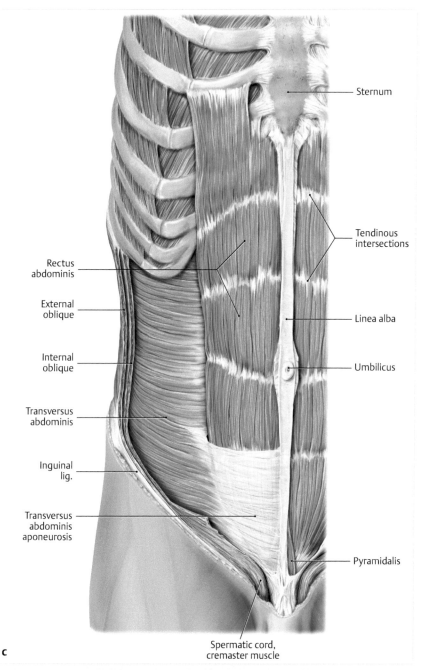

**Fig. 6.4** (*Continued*) **(c)** Deep anterolateral abdominal wall muscles. (Reproduced with permission from Gilroy A, MacPherson B, Schünke M et al., ed. Atlas of Anatomy. 3rd Edition. New York, NY: Thieme; 2017.)

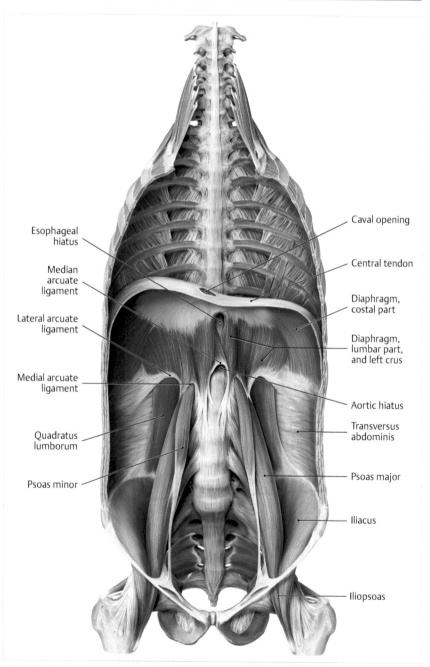

**Fig. 6.5** Posterior abdominal wall musculature. (Reproduced with permission from Baker E, Schünke M, Schulte E et al., ed. Anatomy for Dental Medicine. 2nd ed. New York, NY: Thieme; 2015.)

- Conus medullaris is located at inferior aspect of L1 vertebrae:
  - Spinal cord termination.
- Sympathetic trunk:
  - Bilateral to vertebral column.
  - Connects to anterior rami via rami communicantes.

**Table 6.7** Lumbar vasculature

| Artery | Location | Branches | Supplies |
|---|---|---|---|
| Abdominal aorta | Runs caudally along vertebral canal until bifurcating at L4 | Segmental intercostal arteries Lumbar arteries | Organs and tissues of abdomen, pelvis, and legs |
| Segmental intercostal | Anterior to vertebral bodies and transverse processes Inferior borders of ribs | Dorsal branch Spinal branch Ventral branch Anterior segmental medullary | Dura Spinal cord Vertebral bodies Anterior spinal artery |
| Lumbar | Bilateral arteries Posterolateral along vertebral bodies | Posterior segmental medullary Anterior radicular arteries Posterior radicular arteries | Dorsal back muscles Posterior spinal arteries |
| Anterior segmental medullary | Midline along nerve roots | Anterior spinal artery Anterior radicular arteries | Lumbar and sacral spinal cord |
| Posterior segmental medullary | Paired arteries along nerve roots | Posterior spinal artery Posterior radicular arteries | Lumbar and sacral spinal cord |
| Anterior spinal | Ventral median fissure of spinal cord | Sulcal branches Pial arterial plexus | Anterior two-thirds of spinal cord |
| Posterior spinal | Paired arteries along posterolateral sulci of spinal cord | | Posterior one-third of spinal cord |

**Table 6.8** Lumbar plexus: anterior division

| Nerve | Origin | Motor | Sensory |
|---|---|---|---|
| Subcostal | T12 | | Subxiphoid region |
| Iliohypogastric | T12–L1 | Transversus abdominis Abdominal internal oblique | Above pubis Posterolateral buttocks |
| Ilioinguinal | L1 | | Inguinal region |
| Genitofemoral | L1–L2 | Cremaster | Scrotum (M) Mons (F) |
| Obturator | L2–L4 | External oblique Adductor longus Adductor brevis Adductor magnus Gracilis Obturator externus | Inferomedial thigh |
| Accessory obturator | L2–L4 | Psoas | |

**Table 6.9** Lumbar plexus: posterior division

| Nerve | Origin | Motor | Sensory |
|---|---|---|---|
| Lateral femoral cutaneous | L2–L3 | | Lateral thigh |
| Femoral | L2–L4 | Psoas<br>Iliacus<br>Pectineus<br>Rectus femoris<br>Vastus lateralis<br>Vastus intermedius<br>Vastus medialis<br>Sartorius<br>Articularis genu | Anteromedial thigh<br>Medial leg and foot |

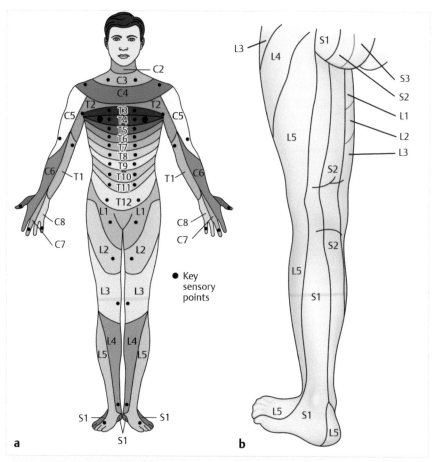

**Fig. 6.6 (a)** Anterior dermatomes. (Reproduced with permission from An HS, Singh K, eds. Synopsis of Spine Surgery. 3rd ed. New York, NY: Thieme; 2016.) **(b)** Dermatomal map of sacral nerve roots. (Reproduced with permission from Baaj AA, Mummaneni PV, Uribe JS, Vaccaro AR, Greenberg MS, eds. Handbook of Spine Surgery. 2nd ed. New York, NY: Thieme; 2016.)

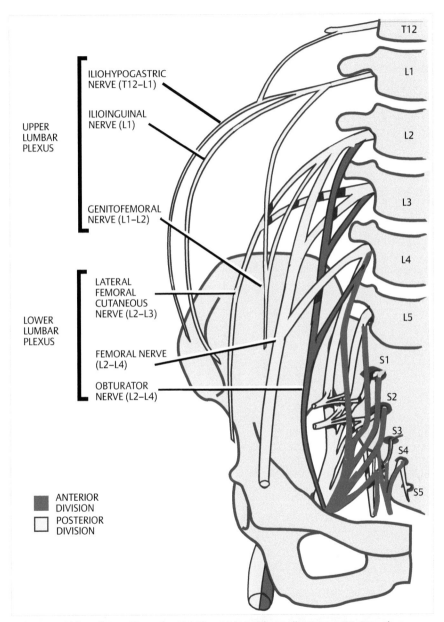

**Fig. 6.7** Lumbar plexus. (Reproduced with permission from Albertstone CD, Benzel EC, Najm IM, Steinmetz M, eds. Anatomic Basis of Neurologic Diagnosis. New York, NY: Thieme; 2009.)

- Lumbar plexus:
  - Anterior rami of T12–L4.
  - Deep to psoas muscle.
- Lumbar dermatomes:
  - Lower back and hips.
  - Anterior, medial, and lateral thighs.
  - Anterior and medial lower leg.
  - Dorsum, medial, and plantar foot.

## Suggested Readings

1.  Gilroy AM, MacPherson BR, Ross LM, Schuenke M, Schulte E, Schumacher U. Atlas of Anatomy. 2nd ed. New York, NY: Thieme; 2012
2.  Drake RL, Vogl W, Mitchell AWM. Gray's Anatomy for Students. Philadelphia, PA: Elsevier; 2005
3.  Thompson JC. Netter's Concise Atlas of Orthopaedic Anatomy. 1st ed. Philadelphia, PA: Elsevier; 2001

# 7 Sacral Spine

*Antonios Varelas, Fady Y. Hijji, Ankur S. Narain, Philip K. Louie, Daniel D. Bohl, and Kern Singh*

## 7.1 General Information

- Begins as five initially unfused vertebrae:
  - Fusion begins around age 18 years and is completed by age 30 years.
- Concave, inverted triangular shape.
- Structural orientation:
  - Base: broad, superior end.
  - Apex: narrow, inferior end.
- Articulations:
  - Ilium: with the superolateral articular surface.
  - L5 (final lumbar vertebrae): with the superior articular process.
  - Coccyx: with the apex of the sacrum.

## 7.2 Bony Anatomy (Fig. 7.1)

- Dorsal (posterior) surface:
  - Contains four pairs of foramina:
    - Allow passage of ventral rami for first four sacral spinal nerves and sacral arteries.
  - Median sacral crest:
    - Fusion of first three or four sacral spinous processes.
    - Bony projection at midline of pelvic surface.
  - Intermediate sacral crest:
    - Fusion of the sacral articular processes of S2, S3, S4.
  - Lateral sacral crest:
    - Fusion of all five sacral vertebral articular processes:
      - Incomplete fusion leads to the formation of the posterior sacral foramina.
- Pelvic (anterior) surface:
  - Four transverse ridges, marking the traces of the four fused intervertebral disks.
  - Sacral promontory:
    - Anterior projection of the pelvic surface.
    - Forms the posterior margin of the pelvic inlet.
    - Less prominent in females than in males:
      - Leads to an oval pelvic inlet in females and a heart-shaped inlet in males.

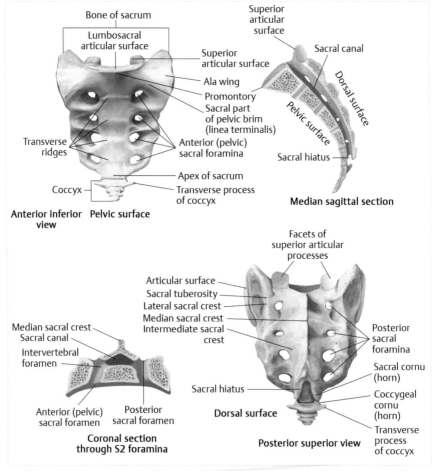

**Fig. 7.1** Bony anatomy of the pelvic, lateral, superior, and dorsal sacral surfaces. (Reproduced with permission from An HS, Singh K, eds. Synopsis of Spine Surgery. 3rd ed. New York, NY: Thieme; 2016.)

- Ala of sacrum:
  - Large superolateral projections of S1 due to fusion of the transverse vertebral processes.
  - L5 nerve root runs over the top of the sacral ala.
- Sacral canal:
  - Inferior extension of the vertebral foramen.
  - Contains the filum terminale and cauda equina:
    - Filum terminale is a nonneural, connective tissue filament that provides longitudinal support for the spinal cord:
      - Fibrous extension of the conus medullaris.

- Filum terminale internum is enclosed within dural sac, while the externum (coccygeal ligament) is extradural and attaches to the first segment of the coccyx.
  - Cauda equina is a collection of spinal nerves and nerve roots of the L1–S5 nerve pairs and coccygeal nerve:
    - Emerges from the conus medullaris.
- Sacral hiatus:
  - An opening at the inferior border of the sacral canal:
    - Occurs when the lamina of the fifth sacral vertebrae fail to fuse.

## 7.3 Ligamentous Anatomy

- Sacroiliac ligaments:
  - Stabilize the sacroiliac joint.
  - Comprises three divisions:
    - Anterior (symphyseal ligaments):
      - Weak stabilization of the sacroiliac joint.
      - Resists external rotation.
    - Posterior (**Fig. 7.2**):
      - Forms the primary bond between sacrum and ilium.
      - Considered by many as the strongest ligaments in the body.
      - Important for pelvic ring stability.
    - Interosseous:
      - Resists abduction of the sacroiliac joint.
- Sacrotuberous ligament (pelvic floor):
  - Spans the sacrum and tuberosity of the ischium:
    - Helps create a boundary for the greater and lesser sciatic foramina.
  - Stabilizes the pelvic girdle.
  - Resists shear and flexion.
  - Passes posterior to the sacrospinous ligament.
- Sacrospinous ligament (pelvic floor):
  - Located within the greater sciatic notch:
    - Spans the sacrum and spine of the ischium.
    - Forms the greater and lesser sciatic foramina.
  - Resists external rotation of the ilium beyond the sacrum.
- Sacrococcygeal ligaments:
  - Spans the sacrum and coccyx.
  - Closes the sacral hiatus.
  - Comprises three divisions:
    - Anterior:
      - A continuation of the anterior longitudinal ligament.

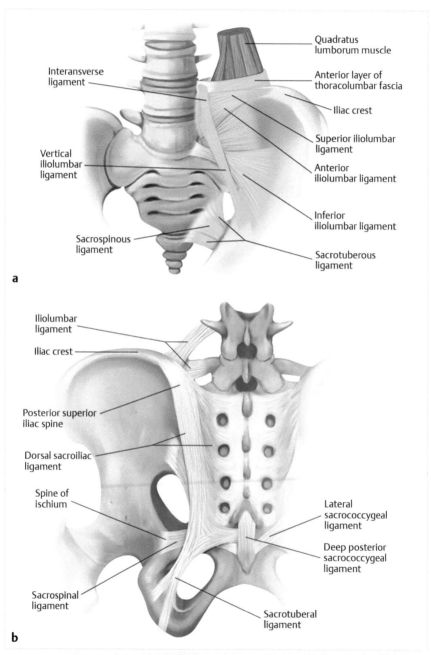

**Fig. 7.2 (a,b)** Posterior views of the sacral ligamentous anatomy. (Reproduced with permission from An HS, Singh K, eds. Synopsis of Spine Surgery. 3rd ed. New York, NY: Thieme; 2016.)

  ○ Posterior:
    ▪ Consists of two components: deep and superficial:
      ❖ Deep ligament is a continuation of the posterior longitudinal ligament.
      ❖ Superficial ligament completes the inferior portion of the sacral canal.
  ○ Lateral:
    ▪ Completes the final foramen for the fifth sacral nerve.
• Coccygeal ligament:
  – Anchors the termination of the dural sac at S2 to the first segment of the coccyx.

## 7.4 Muscular Anatomy

• Anterior sacral muscles (**Table 7.1, Figs. 7.3, 7.4**):
  – Muscular attachments occur along the pelvic (anterior) surface of sacrum:
    ○ Piriformis.
    ○ Coccygeus.
    ○ Iliacus.

**Table 7.1** Anterior surface

| Muscle | Origin | Insertion | Action | Innervation |
|---|---|---|---|---|
| Piriformis | Sacrum (S2, S3, S4) | Greater trochanter of femur | External rotation, abduction, extension of hip joint | Nerve to the piriformis (L5, S1, S2) |
| Coccygeus | Ischial spine, sacrospinous ligament | Inferior sacrum, coccyx | Elevation/support of pelvic floor, flexion of coccyx | Anterior primary rami of S4, S5 |
| Iliacus | Ala of sacrum, iliac fossa | Lesser trochanter of femur | Flexion, external rotation of hip joint | Femoral nerve (L2, L3, L4) |

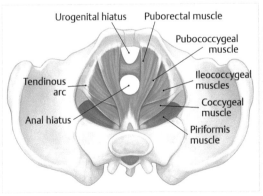

**Fig. 7.3** View of the pelvic floor and the muscular attachments of the piriform and coccygeus to the sacrum.

- Posterior sacral muscles (**Table 7.2, Figs. 7.5, 7.6**):
  - Muscular attachments occur along the dorsal (posterior) surface of sacrum:
    - Multifidus lumborum.
    - Erector spinae.

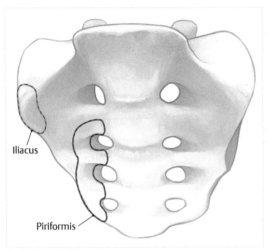

**Fig. 7.4** Anatomical view of the attachment sites for the anterior sacral muscles.

**Table 7.2** Posterior surface

| Muscle | Origin | Insertion | Action | Innervation |
|---|---|---|---|---|
| Erector spinae | Sacrum, iliac crest | Varies for each erector spinae muscle | Extension, lateral flexion of vertebral column and neck | Dorsal primary rami of spinal and thoracic nerves |
| Multifidus lumborum | Sacrum, transverse process of C2–L5 | Spinous processes of vertebrae | Extension, ipsilateral lateral flexion, contralateral rotation of spine | Dorsal primary rami of C1–L5 |

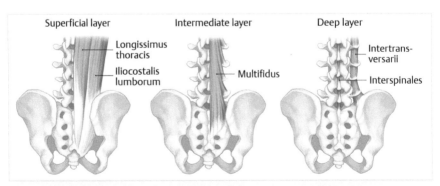

**Fig. 7.5** Posterior view of the muscular attachment of the erector spinae and multifidus lumborum to the sacrum.

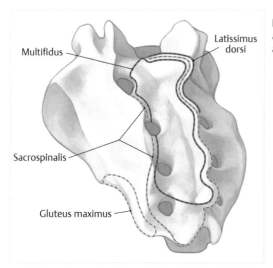

Multifidus

Latissimus dorsi

Sacrospinalis

Gluteus maximus

**Fig. 7.6** Anatomical view of the attachment sites for the posterior and lateral sacral muscles.

**Table 7.3** Lateral border

| Muscle | Origin | Insertion | Action | Innervation |
|--------|--------|-----------|--------|-------------|
| Gluteus maximus | Sacrum, ilium, coccyx | Upper fibers: iliotibial tract<br>Lower fibers: gluteal tuberosity of femur | Extension of hip, external rotation of femur | Inferior gluteal nerve (L5, S1, S2) |

• Lateral sacral muscles (**Table 7.3, Fig. 7.6**):
  - Muscular attachments occur along the lateral edge of sacrum:
    ◦ Gluteus maximus.

# 7.5 Vascular Anatomy

• Median (middle) sacral artery:
  - Vestigial structure.
  - Supplies the coccyx, sacrum, and lumbar vertebrae.
  - Originates from the posterior surface of the abdominal aorta near the aortic bifurcation (**Fig. 7.7**):
    ◦ Descends vertically following the pelvic surface of the sacrum.
    ◦ Terminates in the coccygeal body.
  - Anastomoses:
    ◦ Iliolumbar artery:
      ▪ At the level of the lumbar vertebrae.

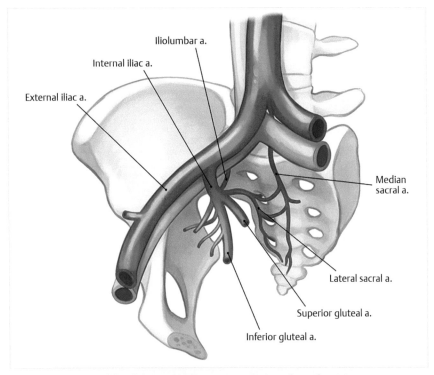

**Fig. 7.7** Anatomy of the abdominal aorta, common iliacs, and sacral arteries.

- Lateral sacral arteries:
  - Anterior to the sacrum.
  - Resulting branches travel through the anterior sacral foramina.
- Lateral sacral arteries:
  - Often observed as bilateral vessels:
    - Superior and inferior.
  - Supply the sacral canal, erector spinae, and piriformis.
  - Originate from the posterior division of the internal iliac artery:
    - Typically manifests as the second branch; however, it can also arise from the superior gluteal artery.
  - Anastomoses:
    - Gluteal arteries:
      - Over the dorsal surface of the sacrum.
    - Median artery:
      - Anterior to the sacrum and coccyx.
    - Contralateral lateral sacral artery:
      - Anterior to the coccyx.

## 7.6 Neural Anatomy

- Nerve roots:
  - Cauda equina contains the sacral fibers (**Fig. 7.8**):
    - Travels within the lumbosacral canal.
    - Collection of L1–S5 peripheral nerves.
    - Dural sac ends at S2:
      - Extradural portion of the filum terminale emerges from dural sac.
  - Upper four sacral roots exit the sacrum by way of the sacral foramina.
  - Fifth sacral root, filum terminale, and coccygeal roots exit through the sacral hiatus.
  - Ventral (anterior) rami of L4–S4 form the sacral plexus.
- Sacral plexus (**Fig. 7.9**):
  - Anterior rami of L4–S3 and the upper portion of S4.
  - Located deep to the pelvic (Waldeyer's) fascia and superior to the surface of the piriformis muscle.
  - Nearly all branches leave through the greater sciatic foramen:
    - Those that remain in the pelvis innervate the perineum, pelvic muscles, and pelvic organs.
  - Gives rise to (**Table 7.4**):
    - Sciatic nerve (L4–S3):
      - Common fibular and tibial nerve components.

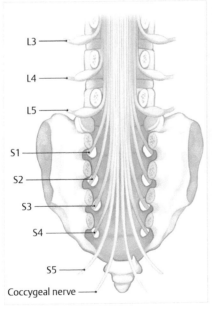

L3
L4
L5
S1
S2
S3
S4
S5
Coccygeal nerve

**Fig. 7.8** Sacral nerve roots passing through the sacral foramina.

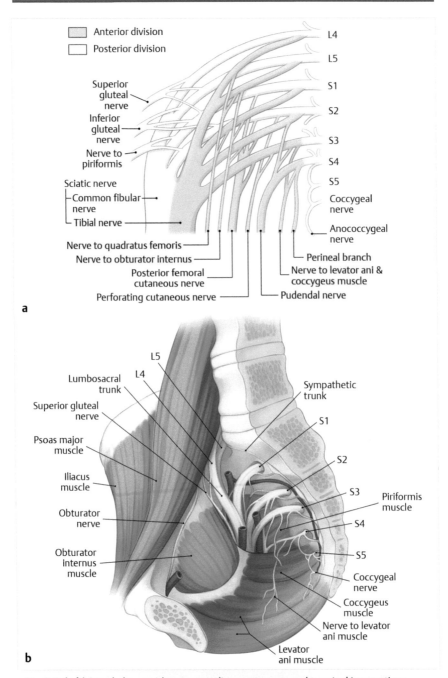

**Fig. 7.9 (a,b)** Sacral plexus with corresponding nerve roots and terminal innervations.

**Table 7.4** Sacral plexus

| Nerve | Origin | Motor | Sensory |
|---|---|---|---|
| Superior gluteal | L4, L5, S1 | Gluteus medius, gluteus minimus, tensor fasciae latae | None |
| Inferior gluteal | L5, S1, S2 | Gluteus maximus | None |
| Nerve to the piriformis | L5, S1, S2 | Piriformis | None |
| Nerve to the obturator internus | L5, S1, S2 | Obturator internus, superior gemellus | None |
| Nerve to the quadratus femoris | L4, L5, S1 | Quadratus femoris, inferior gemellus | None |
| Posterior cutaneous femoral nerve | S1, S2, S3 | None | Perineum, posterior surface of thigh and leg |
| Sciatic | L4, S1, S2, S3 | Tibial portion: semitendinosus, semimembranosus, long head of biceps femoris, adductor magnus (hamstring portion) Common fibular portion: short head of biceps femoris | Tibial portion: posterolateral and medial surface of foot, sole of foot Common fibular portion: anterolateral surface of leg, dorsal portion of foot |
| Pudendal | S2, S3, S4 | External urethral sphincter, external anal sphincter, levator ani, skeletal muscles of perineum | External genitalia, skin of perineum |

- ○ Superior (L4–S1) and inferior (L5–S2) gluteal.
- ○ Pudendal nerve (S2–S4).
- ○ Posterior cutaneous femoral (S1–S3).
- ○ Nerves to piriformis, obturator internus, and quadratus femoris.
- Sacral dermatomes:
  - Sacral nerve roots providing sensation for various areas around the perineum, thighs, and legs.
  - Important dermatomes:
    - ○ S1: posterior thigh and leg (lateral).
    - ○ S2: posterior thigh and leg (medial).
    - ○ S2–S4: perineum and genitals.

# 7.7 Clinical and Surgical Pearls

- Cauda equina syndrome is considered a true medical emergency. Key features include the following: lower extremity sensorimotor changes, bilateral lower extremity pain/weakness, bladder/bowel changes, and/or saddle anesthesia.
- The sacrotuberous ligament is surgically severed to relieve perineal pain resulting from the entrapment of the pudendal nerve between the sacrotuberous and sacrospinous ligament.

- The posterior sacroiliac ligamentous complex are considered the strongest ligaments in the body; they are more important than the anterior ligaments for pelvic ring stability.
- The sacral hiatus offers access to the sacral epidural space for the administration of anesthetics.

## Suggested Readings

1.  An HS, Singh K. Synopsis of Spine Surgery. 3rd ed. New York, NY: Thieme; 2016
2.  Netter FH. Atlas of Human Anatomy. 6th ed. Philadelphia, PA: Saunders; 2014
3.  Herkowitz HN, Garfin SR, Eismont FJ, et al. The Spine. 5th ed. Philadelphia, PA: Saunders Elsevier; 2006:22

# 8 Spinal History and Physical Examination

*Fady Y. Hijji, Ankur S. Narain, Junyoung Ahn, Philip K. Louie, Daniel D. Bohl, and Kern Singh*

## 8.1 Spinal History

### 8.1.1 Background

• Obtaining an accurate clinical history is the most important aspect of evaluation:
  - Physical examination.
  - Diagnostic imaging.
  - Urgency of spinal pathology.
  - Therapeutic modalities.

### 8.1.2 History

• Age:
  - Younger than 40 years: isthmic spondylolisthesis, disk herniation, congenital deformities.
  - Older than 40 years: degenerative disk disease, spinal stenosis, disk herniation.
• Pain:
  - Character:
    ○ Axial versus radicular:
      ▪ Axial: more diffuse/generalized.
      ▪ Radicular (extremities): pain associated with paresthesias, numbness, weakness in a dermatomal distribution.
    ○ Mechanical versus nonmechanical:
      ▪ Mechanical: worse with activity, progresses over the day, relief with rest.
      ▪ Nonmechanical: independent of activity or rest, worse at night.
  - Location:
    ○ Determine anatomic location (neck, back, upper or lower extremity) and presence of radiation:
      ▪ Must distinguish pain due to radiation versus referred pain:
        ❖ Radiating: pain pattern not localizable to a specific dermatome.
        ❖ Referred pain:
          ◇ Shoulder pain referred form cervical spine.
          ◇ Buttocks/posterior thigh pain referred from lumbar spine.
    ○ Determine unilateral versus bilateral nature.

- Timing:
  - ○ Acute: associated with lumbar muscle strain, disk herniation, spondylolisthesis.
  - ○ Progressive: spondylosis, spondylolisthesis, tumor.
  - ○ Night pain: associated with space-occupying lesions (tumors) and infections.
- Alleviating and exacerbating factors:
  - ○ Can distinguish spinal stenosis (neurogenic claudication), disk herniation:
    - ▪ Spinal stenosis improves with sitting, leaning forward:
      - ❖ Vascular claudication differs in that pain is exacerbated by physical activity, pain relief occurs with rest, and weakness is not typically present.
    - ▪ Herniation pain improves with lumbar extension, worse with flexion.
- Mechanism of injury:
  - Trauma: assess airway, breathing, circulation.
  - Activity: often associated with sports.
  - Progressive/atraumatic: common with degenerative conditions.
- Neurologic symptoms:
  - Radiculopathy or neuropathy: paresthesias, numbness, weakness in a dermatomal pattern.
  - Myelopathy: broad-based gait, clumsiness, inability to perform fine motor activities, pain in a nondermatomal pattern.
- Constitutional symptoms:
  - Accompanying fevers, chills, night sweats, and significant weight loss may be consistent with infectious or oncologic etiologies.
- Patient factors that may be associated with spinal pathology:
  - Past medical history:
    - ○ Previous infections, diagnosed tumors, childhood illnesses, neurological diseases.
    - ○ Mental disorders (depression, anxiety) may be associated with low back pain.
    - ○ Underlying systemic illnesses.
  - Family history:
    - ○ Previous history of spinal pathology, spinal tumors, and other cancers.
  - Social history:
    - ○ Inquire about occupation, job satisfaction, previous workers' compensation–related injuries.
    - ○ Recreational activities.
    - ○ Smoking, illicit drug use.

# 8.2  Physical Examination

## 8.2.1  Background

- Physical examination is crucial for narrowing differential diagnoses to identify spine pathology:
  - Must be individualized to patient's presentation:
    - ○ History.

- Anatomic region of suspected pathology.
- Imaging findings.
- Physical examination includes five main components:
  - General:
    - Inspection.
    - Palpation.
    - Range of motion.
    - Walking gait.
  - Sensory.
  - Motor.
  - Reflexes.
  - Special maneuvers.

## 8.2.2  General Physical Examination

- Inspection:
  - Skin:
    - Must disrobe patient adequately for appropriate assessment.
    - Inspect for any unique growths or lesions:
      - Café au lait spots:
        - ❖ Neurofibromatosis.
      - Hair tufts in lumbar region:
        - ❖ Spina bifida.
  - Muscle tone/bulk:
    - Inspect for muscle size or abnormal contractions:
      - Atrophy:
        - ❖ Chronic neuropathy consequently decreasing muscle fiber innervation and usage.
      - Fasciculations:
        - ❖ Neuropathy causing limited innervation of muscle fibers:
          - ◊ Inability to stimulate full muscle contraction.
      - Contractures:
        - ❖ Chronic upper motor neuron pathology causing long-term immobilization and spasticity:
          - ◊ Reorganization of collagen fibers leads to muscles being held in shortened position for extended periods of time.
  - Posture and alignment:
    - Inspect spinal alignment, abnormal bony prominences, and upright position of patient:
      - Malalignment:
        - ❖ Forward-bending test:

◇ Asymmetric ribs or scapulae is often indicative of scoliosis (congenital or degenerative).
❖ Can be associated with abnormal rib and iliac crest prominences.
▪ Neck or pelvic tilting:
❖ Paraspinal muscle spasms:
◇ Consider torticollis in severe neck tilting with pediatric patients or patients taking dopamine antagonist medications.
• Palpation:
  – Soft tissue:
    ◦ Firm palpation of paraspinal muscles to assess for tenderness:
      ▪ Paraspinal muscle tenderness:
        ❖ Can indicate paraspinal muscle spasm, trauma, or myofascial nodes.
  – Bony structures:
    ◦ Firm palpation of spinous processes, sacrum, and coccyx:
      ▪ Spinous process tenderness:
        ❖ Can indicate spinous process fracture.
      ▪ Coccygeal tenderness:
        ❖ Possible fracture or contusion.
• Range of motion:
  – Cervical:
    ◦ Flexion/extension:
      ▪ Chin to chest and occiput to back.
      ▪ Normal flexion: 45 degrees or within 3 to 4 cm of touching chest.
      ▪ Normal extension: 70 degrees.
    ◦ Lateral flexion:
      ▪ Bending ear to shoulder.
      ▪ Normal: 30 to 40 degrees in each direction.
    ◦ Rotation:
      ▪ Turning head in either direction with stationary shoulders.
      ▪ Normal: 70 degrees in each direction.
  – Lumbar:
    ◦ Flexion/extension:
      ▪ Toe touch with straight legs and leaning backward.
      ▪ Normal flexion: 45 to 60 degrees.
      ▪ Normal extension: 20 to 30 degrees.
    ◦ Lateral flexion:
      ▪ Bend at waist to either side.
      ▪ Normal: 10 to 20 degrees in each direction.
    ◦ Rotation:
      ▪ Rotating at the waist with hips stationary.
      ▪ Normal: 5 to 15 degrees.

- Walking gait:
  - Patient walks across examination room.
  - Inspect for abnormal movements or postures:
    - Wide-based gait:
      - Late finding in myelopathy, usually involving the posterior columns of the spinal cord.
    - Leaning forward:
      - Often indicates spinal stenosis.
      - Spinal flexion increases space within spinal canal.
    - Trendelenburg gait (**Fig. 8.1**):
      - Pelvic tilt/drop of the side contralateral to the weight-bearing leg.
      - Indicates hip abductor weakness of weight-bearing side.

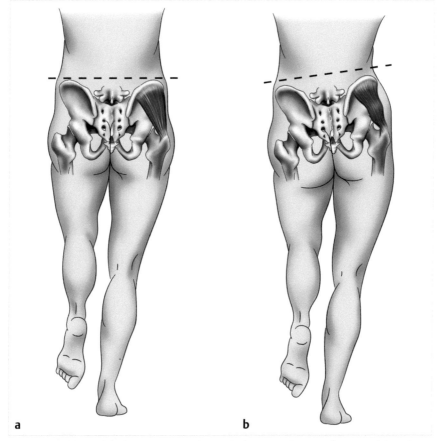

a                                              b

**Fig. 8.1 (a,b)** Trendelenburg gait. Note the weak gluteus medius, resulting in inability of hip abduction of the ipsilateral side.

- Antalgic gait:
    - Shortened stance phase of the walking gait for the side experiencing hip pain.
    - Indicates hip pain/pain with weight bearing.
- Circumduction gait:
    - Excessive leg abduction due to spasticity of leg extensors.
    - Indicates upper motor neuron pathology.
- High-steppage gait:
    - Excessive hip flexion to compensate for foot drop due to weak dorsiflexion.
    - Indicates neuropathy of L4 or L5 nerve root or deep peroneal nerve palsy.

## 8.3  Sensory Examination (Fig. 8.2)

- Four distinct sensory modalities:
    - Pain/pinprick:

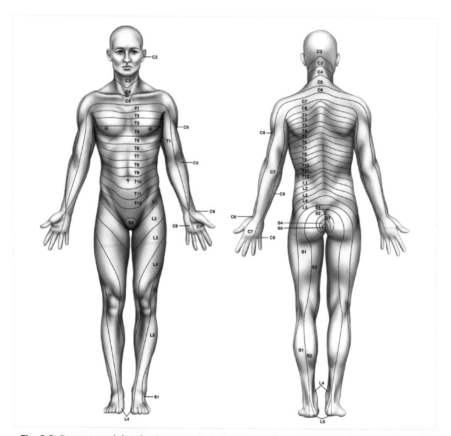

**Fig. 8.2** Dermatomal distribution map. Note that many dermatomes can have overlap with one another.

- Prick patient with slightly sharp object such as a pin or broken wooden cotton swab.
- Assesses nerve root dermatomes and spinothalamic tract.
- Light touch:
  - Gently stroke dermatome with cotton swab or monofilament.
  - Assesses nerve root dermatomes.
- Temperature:
  - Crudely tested using a test tube with hot or cold solution.
  - Assesses spinothalamic tract and status of anterior white commissure.
- Proprioception and vibration:
  - Proprioception: place the patient's big toe in the dorsiflexed or plantarflexed position, and ask the patient to identify its position while their eyes are closed:
    - If they are unable to correctly identify, progressively move to more proximal joints.
  - Vibration sense: place the base of a vibrating tuning fork on the metatarsal phalangeal joint of the big toe and ask the patient to identify the sensation while their eyes are closed:
    - If they are unable to sense the vibration, move to more proximal areas with skin overlying bone (lateral/medial malleolus).
  - Assesses dorsal column of spinal cord.
- Decreased sensation may indicate pathology involving the anatomic pathway of that sensation.

## 8.4 Motor Examination

- Assessment of muscle tone and strength.
- Muscle tone:
  - Resistance to passive range of motion:
    - Move patient arm without any resistance provided by the patient.
    - Assessment must be made at all major joints sequentially:
      - That is, wrist → elbow → shoulder.
  - Hypertonia:
    - Excessive contraction and stiffness to passive movement.
    - Pathology involving upper motor neurons.
  - Hypotonia:
    - No muscular contractions or resistance during passive movement.
    - Pathology involving lower motor neurons.
- Muscle strength:
  - Provide resistance to the muscle being assessed.
  - Five-point grading scale:
    - Grade 5: full strength.
    - Grade 4: weakness against resistance.

- ◦ Grade 3: able to move against gravity but not resistance.
- ◦ Grade 2: able to move perpendicular to gravity, but not against gravity.
- ◦ Grade 1: evidence of contractility (muscle fasciculation).
- ◦ Grade 0: no contractility.
- Decreased motor strength will indicate pathology of either upper (spinal cord) or lower motor (nerve root) neurons:
  - – Muscle tonicity and reflexes helpful in further delineating the type of lesion.

# 8.5  Reflexes (Tables 8.1, 8.2)

- Assessment of the integrity of the entire neural pathway (sensory, central, and motor):
  - – Some reflexes are physiologic, and some are pathologic:
    - ◦ Deep tendon reflex, cutaneous, and sacral reflexes are physiologic.
    - ◦ Babinski's and occasionally Hoffman's reflexes are pathologic.
- Five-point grading scale for deep tendon reflexes:
  - – 5+: sustained clonus.
  - – 4+: hyperreflexic with clonus.

**Table 8.1**  Cervical nerve roots and their predominant sensory, motor, and reflex functions

|  | Sensory | Motor | Deep Tendon Reflex |
|---|---|---|---|
| C5 | Lateral shoulder and arm | Deltoid (shoulder abduction) | Biceps tendon |
| C6 | Lateral arm, forearm and thumb | Biceps (elbow flexion) | Brachioradialis |
| C7 | Index and middle finger | Triceps (elbow extension) | Triceps tendon |
| C8 | Fourth and fifth digits | Hand intrinsics (finger abduction) | – |
| T1 | Medial forearm and arm | Hand intrinsics (finger abduction) | – |

**Table 8.2**  Lumbosacral nerve roots and their predominant sensory, motor, and reflex functions

|  | Sensory | Motor | Deep tendon reflex |
|---|---|---|---|
| L1 | Inguinal crease | Transversus abdominis and internal oblique (trunk flexion) | – |
| L2 | Upper thigh | Psoas (hip flexion) | – |
| L3 | Anterior to medial thigh | Quadriceps (leg extension) | Patellar tendon |
| L4 | Lower anterior thigh and medial leg | Quadriceps and tibialis anterior (ankle dorsiflexion) | Patellar tendon |
| L5 | Posterolateral thigh and lateral leg, plantar foot, first web space | Extensor hallucis longus | Medial hamstrings (rarely used) |
| S1 | Lateral foot, lateral posterior thigh and leg | Gastrocnemius (ankle plantarflexion) | Achilles' tendon |
| S2–S4 | Medial posterior thigh and leg, and perianal region | External and sphincter | Anal wink reflex and bulbocavernosus reflex |

- 3+: slightly hyperreflexic.
- 2+: normal reflex.
- 1+: weak normal.
- 0: no contraction/reflex.
• Hyperreflexia, spasticity, and clonus indicative of upper motor neuron pathology causing poor lower motor neuron inhibition:
  - Hyperreflexia defined as increased brisk reflex with contraction of muscles not directly being assessed:
    ◦ Example: contraction of thigh adductors during patellar tendon reflex.
  - Clonus is involuntary rhythmic muscular contractions and relaxation, often accompanied with spasticity.

# 8.6 Special Maneuvers (Tables 8.3 and 8.4)

**Table 8.3** Cervical tests

| | How to perform | Indicates | Pathologic response |
| --- | --- | --- | --- |
| Spurling's maneuver | Rotate and laterally flex head to one side and then provide an axial load | Compression of a cervical nerve root of the ipsilateral side | Reproduction of a patient's radicular pain |
| L'hermitte's phenomenon | Flex neck toward chin | Compression of the cervical spinal cord | Electrical sensation radiating into back and extremities |
| Grip and release test | Have patient rapidly make a fist and release with both hands | Cervical myelopathy | Patient unable to perform at least 20 cycles of grip/release within 10 s |
| Hoffman's sign | Snapping/flicking patient's distal phalanx of middle finger | Cervical myelopathy (can be normal in young athletes or naturally hyperreflexive patients) | Flexion of distal phalanx of thumb and possibly other digits during maneuver |
| Finger escape sign | Ask patients to fully extend their fingers and maintain this position | Cervical myelopathy | Fourth and fifth digits begin to flex and abduct |

**Table 8.4** Lumbar tests

|  | How to perform | Indicates | Pathologic response |
|---|---|---|---|
| Straight leg raised (SLR) test | With patient supine, flex hip and dorsiflex ankle of the side with radicular pain | Compression of lumbar nerve root | Reproduction of patient's radicular pain at >60 degrees of hip flexion |
| Contralateral SLR | Flex the hip and ankle contralateral to the side of the patient's radiculopathy | Sequestered or large extruded disc herniation | Reproduction of the patient's radicular pain |
| Flip sign (sitting root test) | While patient is seated, distract patient and passively extend knee (assist in putting shoes back on) | True-positive SLR | Pain recreated with knee extension (patient will jerk backward) |
| Romberg's sign | Have the patient stand up with their feet together and eyes closed for 10 s | Posterior column injury | Patient is unable to maintain balance |
| Babinski's sign | Stroke the plantar surface of the patient's foot with a solid mildly sharp object | Upper motor neuron injury or myelopathy (cervical or lumbar) | Upgoing big toe/toes (physiological in infants) |
| Ankle clonus | Rapidly dorsiflex and plantarflex ankle | Upper motor neuron injury or myelopathy | Repetitive beats of clonus |
| Anal wink reflex | Stroke skin around anus to elicit contraction of external anal sphincter | Injury to sacral nerve roots | Absent anal sphincter contraction |
| Bulbocavernosus reflex | Squeeze patient's glans penis or clitoris or tug on indwelling Foley catheter, monitoring for anal external sphincter contraction | Injury to conus medullaris or sacral nerve roots S2–S4 | Absent sphincter contraction |
| Waddell's sign | Thorough history and physical exam | Nonorganic pathology | Four findings: (1) exaggerated responses, (2) pain to light touch, (3) pain in a nonanatomic pattern, and (4) negative sitting root test with positive SLR |

Sustained applied force
*Clonus
Achilles tendon
Soleus muscle
Gastrocnemius muscle

Bulbo-spongious muscle
Percuss glans
External anal sphincter con-stricts

# Suggested Readings

1.  Greenberg MS. Handbook of Neurosurgery. 7th ed. New York, NY: Thieme; 2010
2.  Netter FH. Atlas of Human Anatomy. 6th ed. Philadelphia, PA: Saunders; 2014
3.  An HS, Singh K. Synopsis of Spine Surgery. 3rd ed. New York, NY: Thieme; 2016

# 9 Common Radiographic Measurements

*Dustin H. Massel, Benjamin C. Mayo, William W. Long, Krishna D. Modi, and Kern Singh*

## 9.1 Radiographic Measurements

### 9.1.1 Cervical Measurements (Fig 9.1, Table 9.1)

**Cervical Lordosis**

• Measured via a lateral radiograph.
• May be referred to as a C2–C7 Cobb angle.

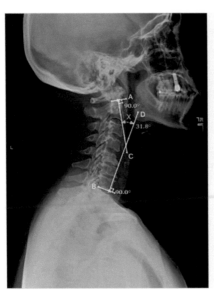

**Fig. 9.1.** Normal cervical lordosis. Line A: drawn in an anteroposterior (AP) direction at the superior end plate of C2. Line B: drawn in an AP direction at the inferior endplate of C7. Line C: drawn in an inferior direction, perpendicular to line A. Line D: drawn in a superior direction, perpendicular to line B. Angle X, measured between lines C and D, represents cervical lordosis.

**Table 9.1** Normal cervical spine curvature measurements (**Fig. 9.1**)

| Spine region | Curvature | Measurements |
| --- | --- | --- |
| Cervical | Hypolordosis | < 20 degrees |
| | Lordosis | 20–40 degrees |
| | Hyperlordosis | > 40 degrees |

## 9.1.2 Thoracic Measurements (Fig 9.2, Table 9.2)

### Thoracic Kyphosis

• Measured via a lateral radiograph.

## 9.1.3 Lumbar Measurements (Fig 9.3, Table 9.3)

### Lumbar Lordosis

• Measured via a lateral radiograph.
• May be referred to as a L1–L5 Cobb angle.

## 9.1.4 Cobb Angle (Fig 9.4)

• Quantifies magnitude of spinal deformities (e.g., scoliosis).
  - Cobb angle ≥ 10 degrees = scoliosis.

For more information on scoliosis, see Chapter 12.

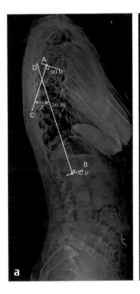
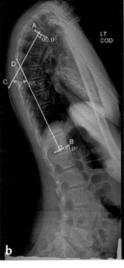

**Fig. 9.2** Thoracic kyphosis. **(a)** Normal thoracic kyphosis. **(b)** Thoracic hyperkyphosis. Line A: drawn in an anteroposterior (AP) direction at the superior endplate of T4. Line B: drawn in an AP direction at the inferior end plate of T12. Line C: drawn in an inferior direction, perpendicular to line A. Line D: drawn in a superior direction, perpendicular to line B. Angle X, measured between lines C and D, represents thoracic kyphosis.

**Table 9.2** Normal thoracic spine curvature measurements (**Fig. 9.2**)

| Spine region | Curvature | Measurements |
| --- | --- | --- |
| Thoracic | Hypokyphosis | < 20 degrees |
| | Kyphosis (**Fig. 9.2a**) | 20–45 degrees (average 35 degrees) |
| | Hyperkyphosis (**Fig. 9.2b**) | > 45 degrees |

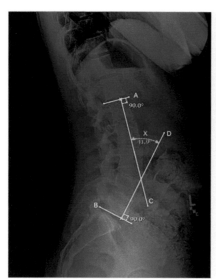

**Fig. 9.3** Normal lumbar lordosis. Line A: drawn in an anteroposterior (AP) direction at the superior endplate of L1. Line B: drawn in an AP direction at the inferior end plate of L5. Line C: drawn in an inferior direction, perpendicular to line A. Line D: drawn in a superior direction, perpendicular to line B. Angle X, measured between lines C and D, represents lumbar lordosis.

**Table 9.3** Normal lumbar spine curvature measurements **(Fig. 9.3)**

| Spine region | Curvature | Measurements |
|---|---|---|
| Lumbar | Hypolordosis | < 40 degrees |
| | Lordosis | 40–60 degrees |
| | Hyperlordosis | > 60 degrees |

## 9.1.5  Coronal Balance (Fig 9.5, Table 9.4)

- Radiograph read as if patient standing with back to you (R on R, L on L).
- **C7 plumb line (C7PL)** = used as a reference to measure displacement of the vertebral bodies from each other and from midline (based on distance from the **central sacral vertical line [CSVL]**).
- **Coronal compensation** = C7 vertebral body directly above the S1 vertebral body (despite abnormal spinal curvature).
- Coronal decompensation = C7 vertebral body laterally displaced from above the S1 vertebral body.

## 9.1.6  Sagittal Vertical Axis (Fig 9.6, Table 9.5)

- Measured via a lateral radiograph.
- Used for cervical sagittal vertical axis (CSVA) or global spine (SVA) measurements.
- **C2 plumb line (C2PL)** = used as a reference to measure displacement of the cervical vertebral bodies from each other and from midline in a sagittal plane:
  - Primary measure of cervical sagittal alignment.

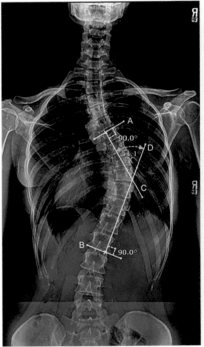

**Fig. 9.4** Cobb's angle. Define upper and lower vertebral levels associated with curvature/deformity. Line A: drawn in an anteroposterior (AP) direction at the superior end plate of the upper vertebral level associated with curvature/deformity. Line B: drawn in an AP direction at the inferior end plate of the lower vertebral level associated with curvature/deformity. Line C: drawn in an inferior direction, perpendicular to line A. Line D: drawn in a superior direction, perpendicular to line B. Angle X, measured between lines C and D, represents Cobb's angle.

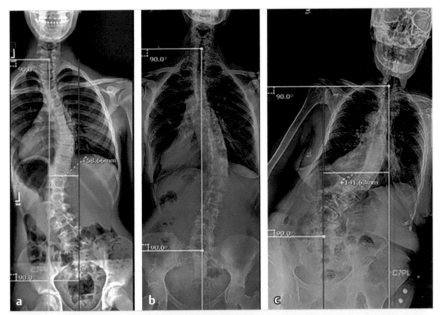

**Fig. 9.5** Coronal balance. **(a)** Negative coronal balance. **(b)** Neutral coronal balance. **(c)** Positive coronal balance. C7 plumb line (C7PL): vertical line drawn from the center of the C7 vertebral body. Central sacral vertical line (CSVL): vertical line drawn from the center of the S1 vertebral body.

**Table 9.4**  Coronal balance (**Fig. 9.5**)

| Figure | Compensation | Coronal balance | Equation |
|---|---|---|---|
| **Fig. 9.5a** | Decompensated | Negative | C7PL – CSVL= – X cm (sacrum to the right of the C7PL) |
| **Fig. 9.5b** | Compensated | Neutral | C7PL – CSVL = 0 cm |
| **Fig. 9.5c** | Decompensated | Positive | C7PL – CSVL = +X cm (sacrum to the left of the C7PL) |

Abbreviations: C7PL, C7 plumb line; CSVL, central sacral vertical line.

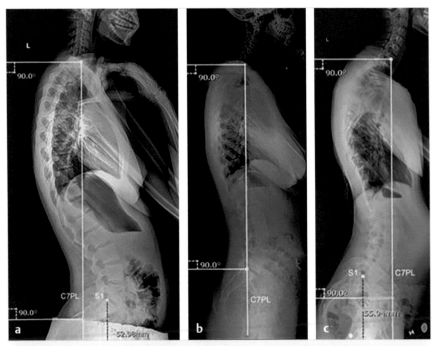

**Fig. 9.6** Global sagittal vertical axis (SVA). **(a)** Negative sagittal vertical axis. **(b)** Normal sagittal vertical axis. **(c)** Positive sagittal vertical axis. C7 plumb line (C7PL): vertical line drawn from the center of the C7 vertebral body. Measure distance from the posterosuperior aspect of S1.

**Table 9.5**  Sagittal vertebral axis (**Fig. 9.6**)

| Figure | Spine region | Sagittal balance | Course |
|---|---|---|---|
| – | Cervical | Negative | C2PL posterior to the PS aspect of C7 |
| – | Cervical | Normal | C2PL runs through the PS aspect of C7 |
| – | Cervical | Positive | C2PL anterior to the PS aspect of C7 (> 40 mm) |
| **Fig. 9.6a** | Global | Negative | C7PL posterior to the PS aspect of S1 |
| **Fig. 9.6b** | Global | Normal | C7PL runs through the PS aspect of S1 |
| **Fig. 9.6c** | Global | Positive | C7PL anterior to the PS aspect of S1 (> 50 mm) |

Abbreviations: C2PL, C2 plumb line; C7PL, C7 plumb line; PS, posterosuperior.

• **C7 plumb line (C7PL)** = used as a reference to measure displacement of the thoracic and lumbar vertebral bodies from each other and from midline in a sagittal plane (in contrast to the C7PL for coronal balance).

## 9.1.7 Pelvic Parameters (Fig. 9.7, Table 9.6)

• Assessed using standing 36-inch lateral radiograph.

| Pelvic rotation | Sacral slope | Pelvic tilt |
| --- | --- | --- |
| Anteversion | High | Low |
| Retroversion | Low | High |

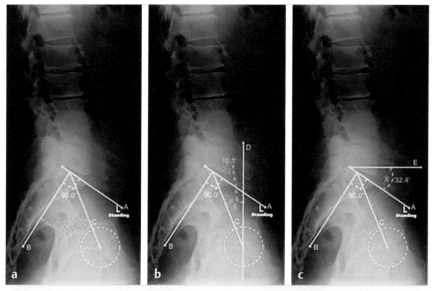

**Fig. 9.7** Pelvic parameters. **(a)** Pelvic incidence (PI). Line A: drawn in an anteroposterior (AP) direction through the sacral end plate. Line B: drawn inferiorly, perpendicular to line A from the midpoint of the sacral plate. Line C: drawn from the midpoint of the sacral plate to the center of the femoral head. Angle X: measures the angle between lines B and C. **(b)** Pelvic tilt (PT). Line A: drawn in an AP direction through the sacral end plate. Line C: drawn from the midpoint of the sacral plate to the center of the femoral head. Line D: vertical line drawn from the center of the femoral head. Angel X: measures the angle between lines C and D. **(c)** Sacral slope (SS). Line A: drawn in an AP direction through the sacral end plate. Line E: horizontal line drawn from the posterosuperior aspect of the sacral plate. Angle X: measures the angle between lines A and E.

**Table 9.6** Pelvic parameters (**Fig. 9.7**)

| Figure | Parameter | Equation | Normal measurement |
| --- | --- | --- | --- |
| **Fig. 9.7a** | Pelvic incidence (PI) | PI = PT + SS | 40–65 degrees; average = 51 degrees |
| **Fig. 9.7b** | Pelvic tilt (PT) | PT = PI – SS | 10–25 degrees; average = 12 degrees |
| **Fig. 9.7c** | Sacral slope (SS) | SS = PI-PT | 30–50 degrees; average = 39 degrees |

Note: PT and SS are inversely correlated.

## 9.2 Radiographic Findings

### 9.2.1 Ankylosing Spondylitis (Fig. 9.8)

• Chronic inflammatory disease of the spine that causes the vertebral bodies to fuse together. Classically causes "bamboo spine."

### 9.2.2 Arthrodesis (Fig. 9.9)

• Fusion of two or more vertebral bodies.
• CT scan arthrodesis is gold standard:

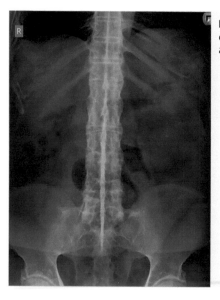

**Fig. 9.8** Anteroposterior (AP) X-ray demonstrating the classic "bamboo spine" appearance of ankylosing spondylitis.

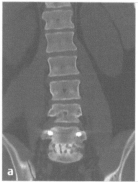 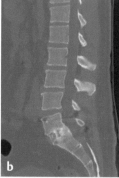

**Fig. 9.9** CT scan arthrodesis. **(a)** Coronal CT demonstrating bony bridging at L5–S1. **(b)** Sagittal CT demonstrating bony bridging at L5–S1.

- Defined by the presence of bony bridging on three sequential cuts in the sagittal and coronal planes.
- The presence of subchondral cysts, end plate sclerosis, or haloing around the interbody cage(s) or pedicle screws are evaluated for possible pseudarthrosis.

### 9.2.3 Pseudarthrosis (Fig. 9.10)

- Nonunion or failed spinal fusion due to inadequate bone formation/bony healing following surgery.

### 9.2.4 Cauda Equina Syndrome

- Severe compression of spinal nerve roots at the end of the spinal cord requiring urgent treatment.

### 9.2.5 Intervertebral Disk Herniation/Herniated Nucleus Pulposus (Fig. 9.11)

- Condition in which the nucleus pulposus is forced through a weakened annulus fibrosus.

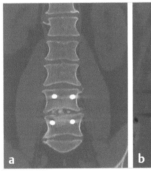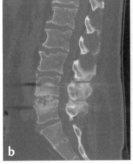

**Fig. 9.10** Pseudarthrosis. **(a)** Coronal CT demonstrating absence of bony bridging at L4–L5. **(b)** Sagittal CT demonstrating absence of bony bridging at L4–L5.

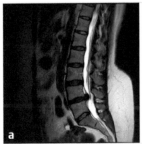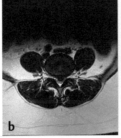

**Fig. 9.11** Intervertebral disk herniation/herniated nucleus pulposus (HNP). **(a)** Sagittal T2-weighted MRI demonstrating HNP at L4–L5. **(b)** Axial T2-weighted MRI demonstrating HNP at L4–L5.

## 9.2.6  Neoplasms of the Spinal Cord

• Tumors located within the spinal cord (extradural and/or intradural).

For more information, see chapter X, page XX.

## 9.2.7  Osteoporosis (Fig. 9.12)

• Condition of reduced bone mass and weakened microarchitecture increasing susceptibility to fracture.

## 9.2.8  Scheuermann's Disease

• Abnormally kyphotic thoracic vertebral alignment.
• Sorenson's classification:
  - Thoracic kyphosis greater than 40 degrees *or* thoracolumbar kyphosis greater than 30 degrees (normal 0 degrees).
  - *And* ≥3 adjacent vertebrae with wedging of greater than 5 degrees.

## 9.2.9  Spinal Stenosis (Fig. 9.13)

• Abnormal narrowing of the spinal canal resulting in compression of the spinal cord (central stenosis) or exiting nerve roots (lateral stenosis).

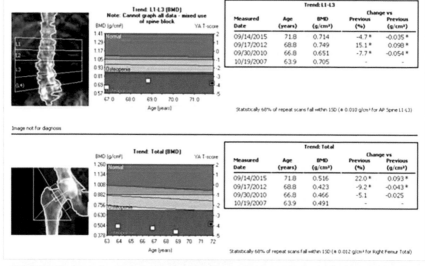

**Fig. 9.12**  Dual energy X-ray absorptiometry (DEXA) scan image of an osteoporotic lumbar spine and right hip. The study includes the L1–L4 vertebral bodies.

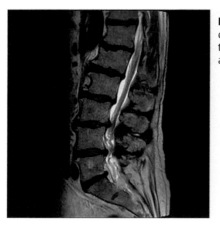

**Fig. 9.13** Sagittal T2-weighted MRI demonstrating significant spinal stenosis as the result of HNP at L2–L3, L3–L4, L4–L5, and L5–S1.

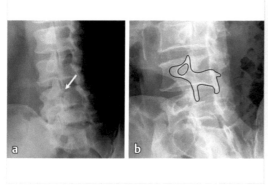

**Fig. 9.14** Spondylolysis. **(a)** "Scotty dog with a collar" on oblique X-ray. **(b)** Outline of the "Scotty dog" on oblique X-ray. The transverse process represents the dog's nose. The pedicle represents the dog's eye. The inferior articular process represents the dog's front leg. The superior articular process represents the dog's ear. The pars interarticularis represents the dog's neck. The contralateral inferior articular process represents the dog's hind leg.

## 9.2.10 Spondylolysis (Fig. 9.14)

• Defect in the pars interarticularis:
  – Associated with isthmic spondylolisthesis.

## 9.2.11 Spondylolisthesis (Fig. 9.15, Table 9.7)

• Anterolisthesis = anterior displacement of vertebral body.
• Retrolisthesis = posterior displacement of vertebral body.
• Classification systems:
  – Wiltse = based on etiology.
  – Meyerding = based on percent slip (most widely used; **Table 9.8**).
  – Marchetti–Bartolozzi = based on etiology (**Table 9.9**).
• Slip angle = quantifies the degree of lumbosacral kyphosis:
  – Slip angle greater than 50 degrees correlates with an increased risk of progression of spondylolisthesis.

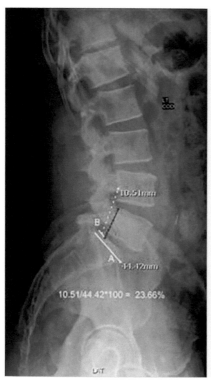

**Fig. 9.15** Measuring spondylolisthesis percent slip. Line A: drawn from the posterosuperior aspect of the nondisplaced vertebrae to the anterosuperior aspect of the nondisplaced vertebrae. Line B: drawn from the posterosuperior aspect of the nondisplaced vertebrae to the posterior edge of the anterolisthetically displaced vertebrae. Divide line B/line A × 100 to determine % slip.

**Table 9.7** Wiltse's classification

| | |
|---|---|
| Type I | Dysplastic (congenital) |
| Type II | Isthmic (acquired) |
| IIA | Lytic |
| IIB | Elongated but intact pars fracture |
| IIC | Acute fracture |
| Type III | Degenerative |
| Type IV | Posttraumatic |
| Type V | Pathologic |
| Type VI | Iatrogenic/postsurgical |

**Table 9.8** Meyerding's classification

| Designation | Grade | Percent slip |
|---|---|---|
| Low grade | I | < 25 |
| | II | 25–49 |
| | III | 50–74 |
| High grade | IV | 75–99 |
| | V | Spondyloptosis > 100 |

**Table 9.9** Marchetti–Bartolozzi classification

| Developmental | High dysplastic | With lysis |
|---|---|---|
| | | With elongation |
| | Low dysplastic | With lysis |
| | | With elongation |
| Acquired | Traumatic | Acute fracture |
| | | Stress fracture |
| | Postsurgical | Direct surgery |
| | | Indirect surgery |
| | Pathologic | Local pathology |
| | | Systemic pathology |
| | Degenerative | Primary |
| | | Secondary |

# 9.2.12 Sacral Inclination (Fig. 9.16)

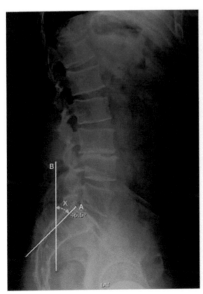

**Fig. 9.16** Measuring sacral inclination. Line A: drawn parallel to posterior aspect of sacrum. Line B: vertical line drawn intersecting line A. Angle X: measure the angle between the posterior aspect of line A and the superior aspect of line B. Normal sacral inclination = 40 to 50 degrees.

# 10 Cervical Disk Disease

*Fady Y. Hijji, Ankur S. Narain, Philip K. Louie, Daniel D. Bohl, and Kern Singh*

## 10.1 Background

- Disk disease is often described as a result of two pathologies:
  - Disk herniation characterized by herniated nucleus pulposus (HNP).
  - Degenerative disk disease (DDD).
- These conditions are common and commonly asymptomatic:
  - 10% of asymptomatic individuals younger than 40 years have HNP on magnetic resonance imaging (MRI).
  - 25% of asymptomatic individuals younger than 40 years have DDD on MRI.
- The progression of a pathologic intervertebral disk may result in compression of adjacent neural structures including the spinal cord and neural roots.

## 10.2 Etiology and Pathophysiology

- HNP:
  - Secondary to stress on annulus of disk:
    - Most often posterolateral as the supportive posterior longitudinal ligament (PLL) is weakest here.
  - Increased risk for herniation from aging and disk degeneration:
    - Decreased water content and proteoglycan content of nucleus pulposus.
  - Characteristics of herniation:
    - Protrusion:
      - Base (neck) wider than head of herniation.
      - Herniation of nuclear pulposus penetrates through annular fibers but remains within the annular margin.
    - Extrusion:
      - Base narrower than head of herniation.
      - Herniation tears through annular margin.
      - Can displace (migrate) cranially or caudally.
    - Sequestration:
      - Free disk fragment separated from original herniation.
- DDD (spondylosis):
  - Aging of disk results in biochemical component changes (**Fig. 10.1**):
    - Decreased cross-linking of collagen, decreased water content.
    - Decreased blood supply to outer annulus:
      - Lactate increases with resultant acidic changes, further degenerating disk.

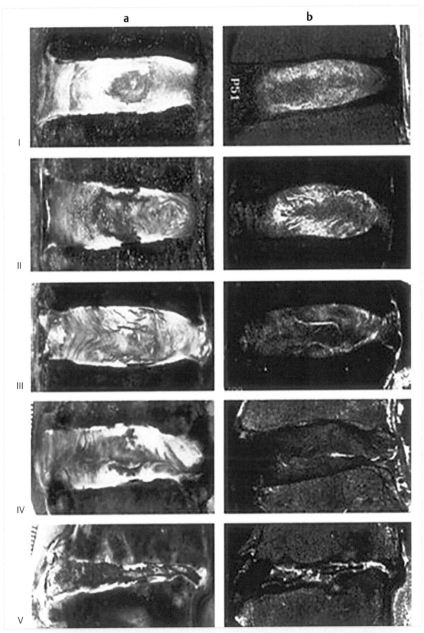

**Fig. 10.1** Thompson disk degeneration staging (I–V). **(a)** Cadaveric examples of disk degeneration with associated **(b)** magnetic resonance imaging for each stage. Note grade I exemplifies characteristics of a healthy disk with appropriate disk height and high water content. Grade V illustrated by significant disk height loss, loss of water content, and bony sclerosis and osteophytes.

- Decreased strength from degenerative changes leads to chronic tears throughout annulus.
- Degenerative cycle includes the following:
  - Disk degeneration (disk bulging, decreased disk space).
  - Joint degeneration (facet arthrosis and uncinate spurring).
  - Ligamentous alterations (ligamentum flavum thickening due to loss of disk height).
  - Spinal deformity (kyphosis, following the loss of disk height and transfer of load to the uncovertebral and facet joints).

# 10.3 Symptoms and Clinical findings (Table 10.1)

- Both DDD and HNP result in tearing of disks with eventual impingement of nearby neural elements including spinal cord.
- Axial neck pain:
  - Unclear etiology.
  - Peripheral disk contains nociceptors and PLL:
    - Annular tears and herniation potentially activates these receptors.
- Radiculopathy:

**Table 10.1** Classification of symptoms resulting from cervical disk disease

|  | Etiology | Symptoms | Physical examination |
|---|---|---|---|
| Axial pain | Inflammation and tears around intervertebral disk | • Central neck pain<br>• With or without referred pain | • Noncontributory<br>• Possible tenderness around paraspinal muscles |
| Radiculopathy | Compression and inflammation of nerve root in the spinal canal or neural foramen | • Radiating pain in dermatomal distribution ± axial neck pain<br>• Numbness/tingling in the in upper extremities<br>• Subjective upper extremity weakness | • ±Spurling's maneuver<br>• ±Shoulder abduction relief<br>• ±Decreased sensation in dermatomal pattern<br>• ±Motor deficit associated with affected nerve root<br>• ±Hyporeflexia |
| Myelopathy | Compression and inflammation of spinal cord within spinal canal | • ±Pain (dull ache to sharp pain)<br>• Difficulty performing fine motor tasks (buttoning a shirt, writing, gripping)<br>• Difficulty walking | • Upper extremity weakness<br>• Glove-distribution sensory loss<br>• Wide-based ataxic gait<br>• Hyperreflexia<br>• ±Hoffman's sign<br>• ±Lhermitte's sign<br>• ±Babinski's sign<br>• Myelopathic hand syndrome (thenar atrophy, decreased dexterity of hands, +grip release test) |

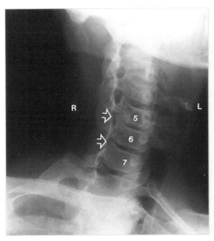

**Fig. 10.2** T1 MRI sagittal and axial views of cervical spine. Note the decreased disk height, disk migration into the cervical canal with canal narrowing, and signal changes within the cord.

- Radiating pain in a pattern consistent with the nerve root involved:
  ○ With or without neurologic symptoms (lower motor neuron symptoms).
- Occurs from direct impingement of nerve roots exiting the spinal cord and vertebral column (**Fig. 10.2**):
  ○ Lateral HNP or osteophytes can compress exiting nerve root near neural foramen:
    ▪ Known as neuroforaminal stenosis.
  ○ Cervical nerve root travels above the similar-named pedicle (i.e., the C5 nerve root travels above the C5 pedicle).
  ○ DDD osteophytes or narrowing of neural foramen, compressing nerve root.
- Inflammation from tears results in chemical radiculitis, furthering radicular symptoms.
• Myelopathy:
  - Upper motor neuron symptoms:
    ○ Patients may present with classic findings:
      ▪ Gait instability.
      ▪ Weakness and clumsiness in manual dexterity.
      ▪ Axial neck pain and stiffness.
      ▪ Diffuse numbness/tingling not isolated to single dermatome.
  - Occurs from central compression of spinal cord:
    ○ Herniation or osteophytic spurs causing narrowing of cervical spinal cord canal (**Fig. 10.2**):
      ▪ Known as central stenosis.
      ▪ Torg–Pavlov ratio: ratio of width of cervical canal to cervical body diameter:
        ❖ <0.8 = central stenosis.
        ❖ Normal is 1.0.
  - Microtrauma from neck flexion/extension along with vascular injury furthers injury to spinal cord.

# 10.4 Imaging

• Plain radiography (anteroposterior [AP], lateral, and flexion and extension views):
  - Initial imaging choice due to cost, ease of access, and ability to evaluate for overall gross pathology.
  - Radiographic findings include the following:
    ◦ Narrowing of intervertebral disk space.
    ◦ Neuroforaminal narrowing.
    ◦ Degenerative changes (osteophytes at end plates or zygapophyseal joints).
  - Visualize alignment on AP and lateral views.
  - Visualize instability/subluxation on flexion and extension views.
• MRI:
  - Imaging of choice for disk disease.
  - Visualize soft-tissue and neurologic structures.
  - Measure space of cervical canal.
  - Can be difficult to distinguish disk from bone.
  - **Correlate with clinical symptoms:**
    ◦ Many asymptomatic patients exhibit degenerative changes.
• Computed tomography (CT):
  - Good for evaluating osseous details, poor for soft-tissue visualization.
  - Requires myelogram to appropriately assess neural pathology:
    ◦ Used when MRI is contraindicated (metal implants, pacemaker) or when time is limited.

# 10.5 Treatment

• Conservative therapy:
  - 70-80% of patients with radiculopathy will improve with conservative therapy.
  - Immediate conservative treatment (initial 2 weeks):
    ◦ Nonsteroidal anti-inflammatory medications.
    ◦ Short-term analgesics. ·
    ◦ Activity modification.
  - Intermediate treatment (3–4 weeks):
    ◦ Physical therapy.
    ◦ Epidural steroids for persistent radicular pain.
  - Rehabilitation (>4 weeks):
    ◦ Physical conditioning.
• Operative therapy:
  - Indications:
    ◦ Continuing or worsening symptoms consistent with nerve root or cord injury.
    ◦ Failure of conservative therapy (typically 3–4 months).
    ◦ Surgery typically avoided for isolated axial neck pain.

- Anterior surgical interventions:
  - ○ Indications:
    - Central disk herniations.
    - Foraminal stenosis.
    - Anterior osteophytes.
    - Spondylotic myelopathy.
- Posterior surgical interventions:
  - ○ Indications:
    - Disk herniation causing radiculopathy.
    - Ossification of the PLL.

## Suggested Readings

1.  Miyazaki M, Hong SW, Yoon SH, Morishita Y, Wang JC. Reliability of a magnetic resonance imaging-based grading system for cervical intervertebral disk degeneration. J Spinal Disord Tech 2008;21(4):288–292
2.  Carette S, Fehlings MG. Clinical practice. Cervical radiculopathy. N Engl J Med 2005;353(4):392–399
3.  Baptiste DC, Fehlings MG. Pathophysiology of cervical myelopathy. Spine J 2006; 6(6, Suppl):190S–197S
4.  Radhakrishnan K, Litchy WJ, O'Fallon WM, Kurland LT. Epidemiology of cervical radiculopathy. A population-based study from Rochester, Minnesota, 1976 through 1990. Brain 1994;117(Pt 2):325–335

# 11 Lumbar Disk Disease

*Fady Y. Hijji, Ankur S. Narain, Philip K. Louie, Daniel D. Bohl, and Kern Singh*

## 11.1 Background

- Axial back pain extremely common:
  - Most common cause is muscle strain, followed by degenerative disease of spine.
- Natural aging and genetic predisposition lead to lumbar disk degeneration:
  - Decreased water content and blood supply to annulus of disk:
    - Results in acidic changes and degeneration of intervertebral disk.
    - After birth, the nucleus pulposus decreases in size and cellularity in proportion to the intervertebral disk.
- Lumbar disk degeneration can result in a mixture of pathologies:
  - Disk herniation characterized by herniated nucleus pulposus (HNP).
  - Spondylosis characterized by degeneration of intervertebral disk and osteophyte formation.
  - Spondylolisthesis characterized by slippage of vertebral body.
- Mean age of onset is 35 years:
  - Over 50% of individuals over 60 years of age exhibit degenerative changes on imaging.

## 11.2 Lumbar Disk Herniation

- Background and etiology
  - 90% of herniated disks occur at L4/L5:
    - Increased risk for herniation from aging and disk degeneration.
  - Chronic or significant acute stress on annulus of intervertebral disk:
    - Leads to annular tears and HNP.
    - Results in direct compression of neural elements.
- Characteristics of herniation *(see Chapter 11: Cervical Disk Disease).*
  - Protrusion:
    - Herniation remains within annular margin.
  - Extrusion:
    - Herniation tears through annular margin but contained by posterior longitudinal ligament:
      - Extends into spinal canal.
      - Can displace cranially or caudally.
  - Sequestration:
    - Separation of herniated disk fragment from intervertebral disk.
- Symptoms and clinical findings:
  - Axial back pain:
    - Controversial etiology.

- Nociceptors along annulus and posterior longitudinal ligament thought to contribute to axial pain with annular tears.
  - Recurrent torsional strain may also lead to outer annulus tears.
  - Worse pain with lumbar flexion in the absence of lumbar spinal stenosis.
- Radiculopathy:
  - Radiating pain in distribution of affected nerve root dermatome:
    - Can be associated with sensory or motor deficits of compressed nerve root.
    - Decreased reflexes of involved nerve root.
  - Herniation impinging of exiting nerve roots:
    - In neuroforamen (neuroforaminal stenosis):
      - Far-lateral herniation.
      - Affects exiting nerve root.
      - Nerve roots exit below pedicle (L4 exits at L4–L5 disk).
  - Herniation of traversing nerve roots (**Fig 11.1**):
    - In spinal canal (spinal stenosis):
    - Paracentral/posterolateral herniation.
    - Affects nerve root traversing to exit at next disk level (L4–L5 paracentral herniation affects L5):
      - Improvement of leg pain with bending forward due to increased space within spinal canal:
        - Known as neurogenic claudication due to the intermittent symptomology.
        - Distinguish from vascular claudication: pain is not relieved by standing still.
- Cauda equina and conus syndromes (**Table 11.1**):
  - Orthopaedic emergencies.
  - Herniation compressing multiple lumbar and sacral nerve roots within the thecal sac or the conus medullaris (T12–L1):
    - Large central herniation.

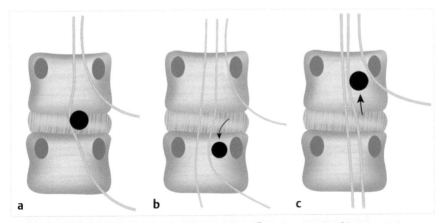

**Fig. 11.1 (a)** Left paracentral L5–S1 disk herniation affecting traversing S1 nerve root. **(b)** Extruded disk L5–S1 herniation migrating inferiorly, compressing the S1 nerve root. **(c)** Sequestered disk herniation migrating superiorly, impinging both L5 and S1 nerve roots.

**Table 11.1** Conus medullaris versus cauda equina syndromes

|  | Conus medullaris syndrome | Cauda equina syndrome |
|---|---|---|
| Vertebral level | L1–L2 | L2 sacrum |
| Spinal level | Sacral cord segment and roots | Lumbosacral nerve roots |
| Presentation | Sudden and bilateral | Gradual and unilateral |
| Radicular pain | Less severe | More severe |
| Low back pain | More | Less |
| Motor strength | Symmetrical, **less marked** hyperreflexic distal paresis of LL fasciculation | More marked asymmetric areflexic paraplegia, atrophy more common |
| Reflexes | Ankle jerks affected | Both knee and ankle jerks affected |
| Sensory | Localized numbness to perianal area, symmetrical, and bilateral | Localized numbness at saddle area, asymmetrical, and unilateral |
| Sphincter dysfunction | Early urinary and fecal incontinence | Tend to present late |
| Impotence | Frequent | Less frequent |

- Imaging:
  - X-ray:
    - Initial evaluation for bony deformities.
    - Often first line for evaluating general degenerative lumbar pathology:
      - Assess for disk space narrowing.
      - Unable to determine disk pathology from plain radiographs.
    - AP and lateral for examining alignment.
    - Flexion/extension for examining instability.
  - MRI:
    - Modality of choice for assessing nerve root or spinal cord compression along with disk and ligamentous pathology:
      - Loss of T2 signal within disk nucleus (**Fig. 11.2**).
    - Modic's changes:
      - Describes vertebral degeneration seen on MRI:
        - ❖ Associated changes on T1- and T2-weighted MRIs with progressive degeneration (**Table 11.2**).
  - Computed tomography (CT) scan:
    - Limited use:
      - If MRI contraindicated.
- Treatment:
  - Conservative therapy:
    - Majority of patients will improve with nonoperative management.

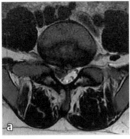
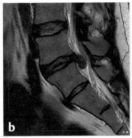

**Fig. 11.2** Axial **(a)** and sagittal **(b)** lumbar T2 magnetic resonance imaging (MRI). Posterolateral disk extrusion of the L5–S1 disk. Note the significant narrowing of the spinal canal and the loss of signal of the posterior disk.

**Table 11.2** Magnetic resonance imaging (MRI) Modic's classification

| Type | Observation | T1-weighted | T2-weighted | Significance |
|------|-------------|-------------|-------------|--------------|
| IU | Normal disk height without dehydration | Hypointensity | Hyperintensity | Bone marrow edema and inflammation |
| II | Normal disk height with dehydration | Hyperintensity | Hyperintensity | Bone marrow ischemia |
| III | Decreased disk height | Hypointensity | Hyperintensity | Subchondral sclerosis |

- ○ Decreasing mechanical stress, maintaining ideal body weight, and smoking cessation all associated with improved outcomes.
- ○ Nonoperative treatment includes rest, physical therapy (PT), anti-inflammatory medication (NSAIDs), muscle relaxants, and oral steroids. 90% of patients improve nonoperatively:
  - Corticosteroid injections are a second line therapy.
- Operative management:
  - ○ Indications:
    - Failure of conservative therapy for at least 12 weeks.
    - Worsening or new onset of neurological deficits.
    - Removal of herniation (microdiskectomy), disk replacement (arthroplasty), or lumbar fusion.

# 11.3 Spondylosis

- Background and etiology:
  - Degeneration of intervertebral disk and articular facets:
    - ○ Broad term to describe osteoarthritic degeneration of the spine:
      - Result of biochemical degenerative changes and chronic stress and pressure.
      - Similar to degenerative process of cervical spine.
  - Osteophytes may form, which may compress neural elements:
    - ○ Osteophytes commonly involve vertebral end plates and articular facets.
- Symptoms and clinical findings:
  - Axial back pain:

- Facet arthropathy thought to be likely cause of pain.
- Worse pain with lumbar extension.
- Radiculopathy:
  - Osteophytic compression of nerve roots:
    - In neuroforamen (neuroforaminal stenosis; **Fig. 11.3**):
      ❖ Facet hypertrophy compressing exiting nerve roots.
    - In spinal canal (spinal stenosis):
      ❖ Posterior end plate osteophytes narrowing spinal canal.
- Cauda equina and conus syndromes:
  - Osteophytic changes resulting in compression of lumbar and sacral nerve roots similar to lumbar herniations.
• Imaging:
  - X-ray:
    - Initial imaging choice to evaluate for overall gross pathology and degenerative changes.
    - Radiographic findings include the following (**Fig. 11.4**):
      - Narrowing of intervertebral disk space.
      - Neuroforaminal narrowing.
      - End plate osteophytes.
      - Facet hypertrophy.
    - Radiographic classification (**Table 11.2**).
  - MRI:
    - Identify compression of neural structures:
      - Bony margins better evaluated on CT.

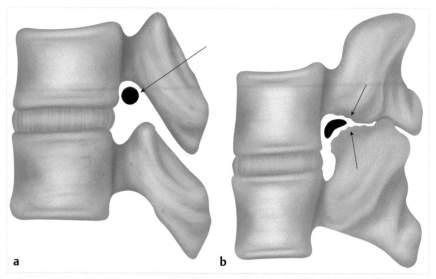

a                                    b

**Fig. 11.3** **(a)** Location of nerve root within the neural foramen. **(b)** Compression of the nerve root due to spondylosis and osteophytes on the superior articular process.

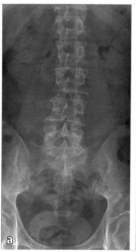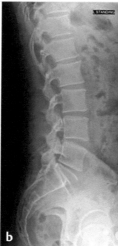

**Fig. 11.4** Anteroposterior **(a)** and lateral **(b)** radiographs. A 50-year-old woman with spondylosis of L5–S1 disk space. Note the neuroforaminal narrowing and loss of disk height.

- Treatment:
  - Conservative therapy:
    - ◦ Similar to conservative management for other lumbar pathologies.
  - Operative management:
    - ◦ Indications:
      - Progressive or new onset neurologic symptoms.
      - Failure of conservative management for minimum of 6 weeks.
    - ◦ Decompression:
      - Laminectomy, foraminotomy, facetectomy.

# 11.4  Spondylolisthesis

- Background/etiology:
  - Anterior or retrograde slippage of a vertebra over the inferior segment:
    - ◦ Often asymptomatic and found incidentally on imaging.
  - 90% of cases occur at L5, 5% at L4, and 3% at L3.
  - Degenerative spondylolisthesis prevalence: 5% in men and 9% in women.
  - Types:
    - ◦ Degenerative:
      - Typically develops after the age of 40 years.
      - Degeneration of facets and intervertebral disk:
        - ❖ Change in stiffness at lumbosacral junction and motion segment instability.
      - Absence of pars defect differentiates these patients from adult isthmic spondylolisthesis.
    - ◦ Isthmic (spondylolysis):
      - Most common among 7- to 20-year-olds.
      - Defect/fracture of the pars interarticularis:

- ❖ Pars interarticularis (between superior and inferior articular processes) susceptible to fatigue and stress fractures:
  - ◊ Cyclic loading of the immature lumbar spine with symptoms occurring later in teenage years.
  - ◦ Congenital/dysplastic, traumatic, and iatrogenic spondylolistheses also occur.
- Classification:
  - Meyerding's classification (**Fig. 11.5**):
    - ◦ Grade I: 25% forward displacement.
    - ◦ Grade II: 25 to 50% forward displacement.
    - ◦ Grade III: 50 to 75% forward displacement.
    - ◦ Grade IV: greater than 75% forward displacement.
    - ◦ Grade V: 100% forward displacement (spondyloptosis).
  - Modified Wiltse:
    - ◦ Based on etiology of the spondylolisthesis (**Table 11.3**).
  - Spinal deformity study group L5–S1 classification (**Fig. 11.6**).
  - Based on pelvic parameters and orientation.

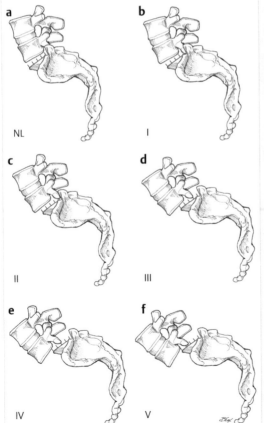

**Fig. 11.5** Meyerding's classification. **(a)** Normal.
**(b)** Grade I, 0 to 25%.
**(c)** Grade II, 26 to 50%.
**(d)** Grade III, 51 to 75%.
**(e)** Grade IV, 76 to 100%.
**(f)** Grade V, spondyloptosis.

**Table 11.3** Spondylosis grading

| Grade 0 | Grade 1 | Grade 2 | Grade 3 | Grade 4 |
|---|---|---|---|---|
| Normal healthy spine | Minimal anterior osteophyte formation | Anterior osteophyte formation | Anterior osteophyte formation | Large osteophyte formation |
| | No reduction in intervertebral (IV) disk height, no vertebral end plate sclerosis | Subtle reduction in IV disk height | Moderate narrowing of disk space | Severe disk plate narrowing |
| | | Subtle sclerosis of endplates | Define sclerosis of endplates, and osteophyte sclerosis | Sclerosis endplate with irregularities |

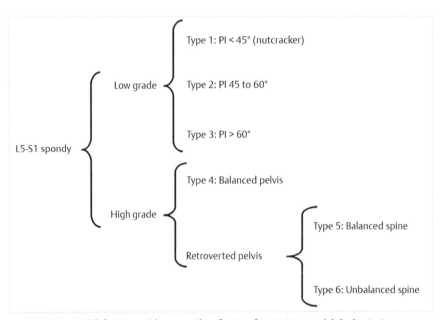

**Fig. 11.6** Spinal deformity study group classification for L5–S1 spondylolisthesis. PI, pelvic incidence.

- Types 1 and 2 exhibit lower risk of disease progression.
  - Higher types (types 5 and 6) indicative of surgical reduction.
- Symptoms and clinical findings:
  - Axial back pain:
    - Little to no back pain as a result of spondylolisthesis alone:
      - Associated degenerative processes (HNP, spondylosis) can cause concurrent pain.

- Radiculopathy:
  - ◦ Experienced by 50% of patients.
  - ◦ Narrowing of spinal canal and neuroforamen due to slippage of vertebral body:
    - ▪ Compression of traversing nerve roots.
- Neurogenic claudication:
  - ◦ May be unilateral or bilateral.
  - ◦ Buttock and leg pain/discomfort caused by upright walking; relieved by sitting.
  - ◦ Not relieved by standing in one place (vs. vascular claudication).
- Cauda equina and conus syndromes:
  - ◦ Similar to other pathologies resulting in compression of lumbar and sacral nerve roots.
- Imaging:
  - X-ray:
    - ◦ Assessment of degree of spondylolisthesis as well as other degenerative processes.
    - ◦ Identify isthmic spondylolisthesis:
      - ▪ Defect in pars interarticularis ("Scottie dog" projection); best evaluated on oblique views.
    - ◦ Slip angle (**Fig. 11.7**):
      - ▪ Angle between superior end plate of L5 and a perpendicular line through the posterior border of the sacrum.
      - ▪ Provides indication of potential stability:
        - ❖ Surgical reduction involves correction of slip angle and resulting lumbosacral kyphosis:
          - ◊ Complete reduction not crucial for clinical success, and actually involves significant risks.
          - ◊ Improves surgical fusion rate.
    - ◦ Flexion–extension views (**Fig. 11.8**):
      - ▪ Identifies lumbar instability.
      - ▪ Greater than 4 mm or 10 of vertebral motion is indicative of dynamic instability.

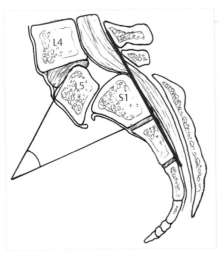

**Fig. 11.7** Slip angle in spondylolisthesis. Angle is formed between the line parallel to superior end plate of L5 and line perpendicular to posterior border of sacrum. (Reproduced with permission from Anderson D, Vaccaro A, eds. Decision Making in Spinal Care. 2nd ed. New York, NY: Thieme; 2012.)

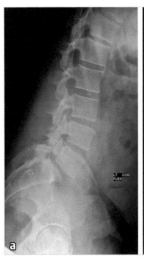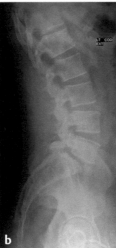

**Fig. 11.8 (a,b)** Flexion-extension radiographic views. Grade 1 L5–S1 isthmic spondylolisthesis. Note the anterolisthesis of the L5 vertebrae over the sacrum with a defect in the pars interarticularis of L5.

- MRI:
  ○ Evaluation of compression of neural structures from slipping vertebral disk.
- Treatment:
  - Conservative therapy:
    ○ Similar to other pathologies causing compression of neural structures.
  - Operative:
    ○ Indications:
      ▪ Persistent or worsening neurologic symptoms.
      ▪ High-grade slippage in the setting of pain or radicular symptoms.
    ○ Lumbar decompression and instrumented fusion:
      ▪ Posterior approach is most common.
      ▪ Decompression via laminectomy.
    ○ Lumbar decompression alone: only recommended for patients that cannot tolerate instrumentation:
      ▪ 31% percent of patients have progressive instability.

## Suggested Readings

1. Baaj AA, Mummaneni PV, Uribe JS, Vaccaro AR, Greenburg MS. Handbook of Spine Surgery. 2nd ed. New York, NY: Thieme; 2016
2. Boden SD. The Aging Spine: Essentials of Pathophysiology, Diagnosis, and Treatment. Philadelphia, PA: WB Saunders; 1991
3. Brier SR. Primary Care Orthopedics. St. Louis, MO: Mosby; 1999
4. Derek M. Degenerative spondylolisthesis. Orthobullets. N.p., June 25, 2016. Web. July 31, 2016

5.  Derek M. Lumbar disc herniation. Orthobullets. N.p., June 11, 2016. Web. July 31, 2016

6.  Ofiram E, Garvey TA, Schwender JD, et al. Cervical degenerative index: a new quantitative radiographic scoring system for cervical spondylosis with interobserver and intraobserver reliability testing. J Orthop Traumatol 2009;10(1):21–26

7.  Winkel D, Vleeming A. eds. Diagnosis and Treatment of the Spine: Nonoperative Orthopaedic Medicine and Manual Therapy. Austin, TX: Pro-ed; 2003

# 12 Scoliosis

*Lauren M. Sadowsky, Ankur S. Narain, Fady Y. Hijji, Philip K. Louie, Daniel D. Bohl, and Kern Singh*

## 12.1 Introduction

Spinal deformities such as scoliosis represent some of the most challenging cases for spinal surgeons. Scoliosis has a variety of potential etiologies, and progresses in severity from childhood to adulthood. Significant functional and cosmetic deficits can occur without proper screening, diagnosis, and treatment of this disorder. As such, it is important to understand the unique clinical history, radiographic techniques and measurement, and surgical strategies that present or are utilized in cases of scoliosis.

## 12.2 Background and Etiology

- Scoliosis is defined as a lateral curvature of the spine ≥10 degrees, typically accompanied with a variable degree of vertebral rotation.
- Etiologies include idiopathic (80–85%), congenital, neuromuscular, and syndromic:
  - Idiopathic:
    ○ Categorized based on age of presentation:
      ▪ Infantile: 0 to 3 years.
      ▪ Juvenile: 4 to 10 years.
      ▪ Adolescent: 11 to 17 years.
      ▪ Adult: ≥18 years (after skeletal maturity).
  - Congenital:
    ○ Present at birth.
    ○ Can include failure of formation (e.g., hemivertebra) or failure of segmentation (e.g., congenital fusion):
      ▪ Often associated with genitourinary deformities.
  - Neuromuscular:
    ○ Due to muscular tone abnormalities (imbalance and lack of trunk control):
      ▪ Etiologies include cerebral palsy, myelomeningocele, myopathies, spinal cord trauma, and muscular dystrophies.
  - Syndromic:
    ○ Includes any syndrome presenting with scoliosis that is not neuromuscular or congenital:
      ▪ Associated syndromes include Marfan's syndrome, osteogenesis imperfecta, skeletal dysplasias, Prader–Willi syndrome, Ehler–Danlos syndrome, and neurofibromatosis.
- Risk factors for acquired scoliosis:
  - 2-4% of all adolescents have adolescent idiopathic scoliosis (AIS):
    ○ Females and males affected equally.

- ◦ Risk of curve progression affects females 10 times more than males:
  - ▪ Larger Cobb's angles in females than in males.
- – Genetics: 97% of AIS patients have a family history of scoliosis.
- – Age: up to 68% of adults older than 60 years have scoliosis due to progression of degenerative changes of the spine.
- • Progression of deformity:
  - – Physiologic changes due to compressive forces on intervertebral disks and vertebrae on concave side → reduced growth and continued asymmetry.

# 12.3 History and Clinical Findings

- • History:
  - – Age at onset:
    - ◦ Peak growth occurs in males at 13.5 years and in females at 11.5 years.
    - ◦ Scoliosis may progress during peak growth spurt.
  - – Presence of back pain and stiffness:
    - ◦ 23% of AIS patients present with pain.
  - – Muscle fatigue from muscle strain and compensated posture.
  - – Shortness of breath/difficulty breathing due to severe thoracic scoliosis.
  - – Family history:
    - ◦ Incidence increases seven times with a first-degree relative with scoliosis.
- • Inspection:
  - – Any truncal imbalance in height/symmetry of shoulders, scapulae, spine, and waistline.
  - – Head misaligned over sacrum (trunk shift).
  - – Findings suggestive of other diagnoses: café au lait spots (neurofibromatosis type 1), axillary freckling (neurofibromatosis type 1), and hair tufts (spina bifida).
  - – Sexual maturity measured by Tanner's grading stages.
- • Height measurement:
  - – Monitor progression and skeletal growth.
- • Adams' forward bend test (**Fig. 12.1**):
  - – Patient bends forward until waist is 90 degrees.
  - – Positive findings include unilateral prominence (thoracic or lumbar), rotational deformity, misaligned shoulders/hips, and asymmetry.
  - – Specific for rotational component of scoliosis.
- • Scoliometer measurements:
  - – Obtained successively during the Adams' forward bend test at three areas of interest both standing and sitting:
    - ◦ Upper thoracic (T3–T4).
    - ◦ Main thoracic (T5–T12).
    - ◦ Thoracolumbar (T12–L1 or L2–L3).
  - – Measurements ≠ 0 are abnormal and define asymmetry.
- • Pelvic tilt:
  - – Lateral pelvic tilt is associated with compensation for scoliosis or leg length discrepancy.
  - – Sagittal pelvic tilt is associated with compensation for curve deformities.

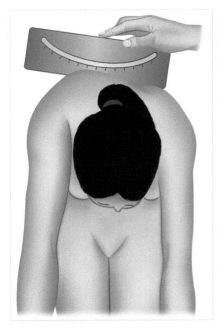

**Fig. 12.1** Adams' forward bend test with scoliometer measurements. (Reproduced with permission from Albert TJ, Vaccaro, AR, eds. Physical Examination of the Spine. 2nd ed. New York, NY: Thieme; 2016.)

- Neurologic examination:
  - Deficits may include abnormalities of gait and coordination, sensory changes, weakness, or incontinence.
  - Presence of neurological symptoms may suggest etiologies other than idiopathic.

# 12.4 Imaging

- Plain radiography:
  - Initial evaluation with standing posteroanterior (PA) and lateral views from the cervical to sacral regions:
    ◦ Determination of curve patterns:
      ▪ Curve direction is determined by convexity:
        ❖ Major curve: largest.
        ❖ Minor curve: smaller.
    ◦ Identification of apical vertebral:
      ▪ Most laterally deviated vertebra from the vertical axis.
    ◦ Determination of the central sacral vertical line (CSVL):
      ▪ Vertical line drawn from the center of the sacrum.
- Cobb's angle:
  - Measured from the proximal and distal end vertebrae of each curve.
  - Measurement protocol:
    ◦ Identify the end plates of the associated end vertebrae.
    ◦ Draw a parallel line extending from each end plate.

- Draw a line at 90 degrees to each parallel line.
  - The angle of intersection for those lines = Cobb's angle.
- Risser's sign:
  - Measures skeletal maturity based on the degree of iliac apophysis ossification on PA radiographs:
    - Grade 0: no ossification.
    - Grade 1: less than 25% ossification.
    - Grade 2: 25 to 50% ossification.
    - Grade 3: 50 to 75% ossification.
    - Grade 4: 75 to 100% ossification.
    - Grade 5: full bony fusion of apophysis to ileum.
  - Lower Risser's grade = greater risk for curve progression.
- Neutral and stable vertebrae:
  - Neutral vertebrae = vertebrae without axial rotation (not within a curve).
  - Stable vertebrae = vertebrae most closely bisected by the CSVL (within a curve).
- Plumb line:
  - Vertical line drawn inferiorly from the midpoint of C7.
  - Measures coronal balance (with AP radiographs):
    - Determine distance between CSVL and plumb line.
  - Measures sagittal balance (with lateral radiographs):
    - Determine distance between posterosuperior S1 and plumb line.
  - Abnormal finding (for both coronal and sagittal balance measurements) is distance greater than 2 cm.
- Lenke's classification system (**Fig. 12.2**):
  - Standing anteroposterior (AP), standing lateral, and right- and left-bending PA radiographs required.
  - Classification includes three components: (1) curve type, (2) lumbar spine modifier, and (3) thoracic sagittal modifier:
    - Curve type:
      - Based on location of curve apices and curve type:
      - Major curve: largest Cobb's angle, structural:
        ❖ Structural curves have greater than 25-degree Cobb's angle on AP side-bending views.
      - Minor curves: all other angles, structural or nonstructural.
    - Lumbar spine modifier:
      - Based on location of CSVL in relation to lumbar curve apex.
    - Thoracic sagittal modifier:
      - Based on the angle of thoracic (T5–T12) kyphosis.
  - Lenke's classification helps guide management, specifically denoting levels of fusion with operative treatment.

# 12.5 Treatment

- Factors to consider for surgical decision making:
  - Degree and type of deformity:

**Curve Type**

| Type | Proximal Thoracic | Main Thoracic | Thoracolumbar / Lumbar | Curve Type |
|------|-------------------|---------------|------------------------|------------|
| 1 | Nonstructural | Structural (major) | Nonstructural | Main thoracic (MT) |
| 2 | Nonstructural | Structural (major) | Nonstructural | Double thoracic (DT) |
| 3 | Nonstructural | Structural (major) | Structural | Double major (DM) |
| 4 | Structural | Structural (major) | Structural | Triole major (TM) |
| 5 | Nonstructural | Nonstructural | Structural (major) | Thoracolumbar / lumbar (TL/L) |
| 6 | Nonstructural | Structural | Structural (major) | Thoracolumbar / lumbar structural MT |

**Structural Criteria**

Proximal thoracic: - Side bending cobb ≥ 25°
  - T2 – T5 kyphosis ≥ + 20°

Main thoracic : Side bending cobb ≥ 25°

Thoracolumbar / lumbar : - Side bending cobb ≥ 25°
  - T10 – L2 kyphosis ≥ + 20°

**Location of Apex (SRS definition)**

| Curve | Apex |
|-------|------|
| Thoracic | T2 – T11–12 DISC |
| Thoracolumbar | T2 – L1 |
| Lumbar | L1–2 DISC – L4 |

**Modifiers**

| Lumbar Spino Modifier | CSVL to Lumbar Apox |
|------------------------|----------------------|
| A | CSVL between pedicles |
| B | CSVL touches apical body(ies) |
| C | CSVL completely medical |

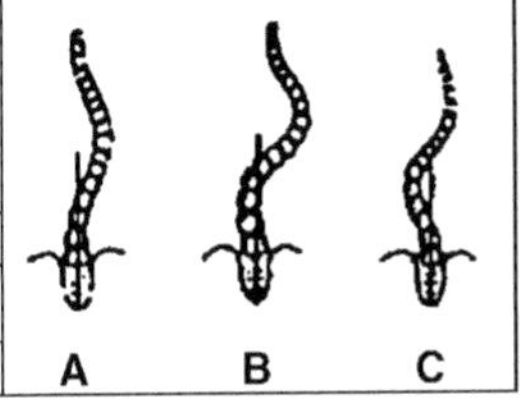

A    B    C

| Thoracic Sagittal Profile T5 - T12 | | |
|---|---|---|
| – | (hypo) | < 10° |
| N | (normal) | 10°-40° |
| + | (hyper) | > 40° |

Curve type (1-6) + Lumbar spine modifier (A, B, or C) + Thoracic sagittal modifier (–, N, or +)
Classification (e.g. 1B+): _____

**Fig. 12.2** Lenke's classification system. (Reproduced with permission from Lenke LG, Betz RR, Harms J, et al. Adolescent idiopathic scoliosis: a new classification to determine extent of spinal arthrodesis. J Bone Joint Surg Am 2001;83-A:1169- 1181.)

- ○ Cobb's angle.
- ○ Radiographic measurements: cervical lordosis, thoracic kyphosis, lumbar lordosis, coronal balance, sagittal vertical axis, pelvic incidence, pelvic tilt, and sacral slope (see Chapter 9).
- Risk for curve progression (Risser's sign).
- Patient maturity and concerns for cosmesis.
• Nonoperative treatment:
- Observation:
  - ○ Cobb's angle of less than 20 degrees.
  - ○ Requires radiographic monitoring every 6 to 12 months.
- Orthosis:
  - ○ A 20- to 40-degree Cobb's angle.
  - ○ Monitoring of progression:
    - ▪ Twenty to thirty degrees initially → start bracing when progression is greater than 5 degrees between consecutive visits.

- Thirty to forty-five degrees initially with Risser's grade ≤ 2 → start bracing at first visit.
  - Thoracolumbosacral orthosis (TLSO) braces:
    - Full-time wear braces.
    - Wilmington brace (total contact TLSO):
      - ❖ Custom-fitted plastic jacket.
      - ❖ Corrects curves with apices at or below T7.
    - Boston brace ("underarm" brace):
      - ❖ Prefabricated sizes modified to individual patients.
      - ❖ Indicated for cervicothoracic, thoracic, thoracolumbar, and lumbar curves.
  - Nighttime braces:
    - Indicated for flexible, single structural thoracolumbar and lumbar curves.
    - Charleston brace ("side-bending" orthosis):
      - ❖ Custom-fitted to provide an "overcorrected" position.
    - Providence brace:
      - ❖ Computer-assisted design brings apices toward vertical axis.
  - Flexible braces:
    - SpineCor brace:
      - ❖ A Cobb angle of ≥15 degrees, full-time wear.
      - ❖ Indicated for single structural thoracolumbar and lumbar curves.
      - ❖ Plastic pelvic base with cotton/elastic corrective bands.
- Operative treatment (**Fig. 12.3**):
  - A Cobb angle of ≥45 to 50 degrees.
  - Indications include failure of conservative therapy, disabling pain, or imbalance.
  - Spinal fusion with instrumentation:
    - Intended to prevent or control curve progression.
    - Anterior and posterior surgical approaches:
      - All major and structural minor curves should be included in the fusion.
      - Neutral/stable vertebrae mark the limits of fusion.

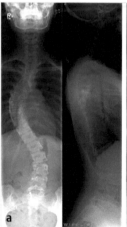 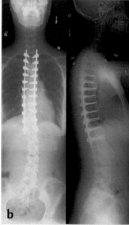

**Fig. 12.3 (a)** Preoperative anteroposterior and lateral radiographs demonstrating significant right thoracic and left lumbar scoliosis. **(b)** Postoperative anteroposterior and lateral radiographs demonstrating correction via fusion with posterior instrumentation.

- Posterior fusion with instrumentation (combination of rods, hooks, and pedicle screws) is the gold standard.
  - Anterior fusion may allow for better results with shorter fusion segments.
- Growth-friendly options:
  - Indications include potential for axial growth, deformity of greater than 50-degree Cobb's angle, and flexible spinal column.
  - Serial casting (every 8–16 weeks).
  - Distraction-based implants:
    ○ Growing rods.
    ○ Vertical expandable prosthetic titanium rib (VEPTR).
    ○ Guided-growth implants.
    ○ Compression-based implants.

## Suggested Readings

1. Abbassi V. Growth and normal puberty. Pediatrics 1998;102(2, Pt 3):507–511
2. Cassar-Pullicino VN, Eisenstein SM. Imaging in scoliosis: what, why and how? Clin Radiol 2002;57(7):543–562
3. Fayssoux RS, Cho RH, Herman MJ. A history of bracing for idiopathic scoliosis in North America. Clin Orthop Relat Res 2010;468(3):654–664
4. Gomez JA, Lee JK, Kim PD, Roye DP, Vitale MG. "Growth friendly" spine surgery: management options for the young child with scoliosis. J Am Acad Orthop Surg 2011;19(12):722–727
5. Horne JP, Flannery R, Usman S. Adolescent idiopathic scoliosis: diagnosis and management. Am Fam Physician 2014;89(3):193–198
6. Janicki JA, Alman B. Scoliosis: review of diagnosis and treatment. Paediatr Child Health 2007;12(9):771–776
7. Kim H, Kim HS, Moon ES, et al. Scoliosis imaging: what radiologists should know. Radiographics 2010;30(7):1823–1842
8. Konieczny MR, Senyurt H, Krauspe R. Epidemiology of adolescent idiopathic scoliosis. J Child Orthop 2013;7(1):3–9
9. Lonstein JE, Carlson JM. The prediction of curve progression in untreated idiopathic scoliosis during growth. J Bone Joint Surg Am 1984;66(7):1061–1071
10. Lonstein JE. Adolescent idiopathic scoliosis. Lancet 1994;344(8934):1407–1412
11. Miller NH. Cause and natural history of adolescent idiopathic scoliosis. Orthop Clin North Am 1999;30(3):343–352, vii
12. Panchmatia JR, Isaac A, Muthukumar T, Gibson AJ, Lehovsky J. The 10 key steps for radiographic analysis of adolescent idiopathic scoliosis. Clin Radiol 2015;70(3):235–242
13. Patias P, Grivas TB, Kaspiris A, Aggouris C, Drakoutos E. A review of the trunk surface metrics used as scoliosis and other deformities evaluation indices. Scoliosis 2010;5(12):12
14. Reamy BV, Slakey JB. Adolescent idiopathic scoliosis: review and current concepts. Am Fam Physician 2001;64(1):111–116

15. Schiller JR, Thakur NA, Eberson CP. Brace management in adolescent idiopathic scoliosis. Clin Orthop Relat Res 2010;468(3):670–678
16. Walker AP, Dickson RA. School screening and pelvic tilt scoliosis. Lancet 1984;2(8395):152–153
17. Wynne-Davies R. Familial (idiopathic) scoliosis. A family survey. J Bone Joint Surg Br 1968;50(1):24–30
18. Yang S, Andras LM, Redding GJ, Skaggs DL. Early-onset scoliosis: a review of history, current treatment, and future directions. Pediatrics 2016;137(1)

# 13 Spinal Trauma and Fractures

*Ankur S. Narain, Fady Y. Hijji, Philip K. Louie, Daniel D. Bohl, and Kern Singh*

## 13.1 General Principles

- Background:
  - Cervical injury occurs in 2 to 3% of blunt trauma cases.
  - Thoracolumbar injury represents 75 to 90% of spinal trauma.
  - Sacral fractures often present with pelvic injuries (30–45%).
- Initial management:
  - Primary survey and neurologic assessment:
    - ABCDE: **A**irway, **B**reathing, **C**irculation, **D**isability, **E**xposure.
  - Secondary survey:
    - Evaluate for spinal shock: check bulbocavernosus reflex:
      - Intact if anal sphincter contraction is observed in response to squeezing the glans penis or pulling on a Foley catheter.
    - Evaluate for neurologic shock:
      - Loss of sympathetic tone leads to circulatory collapse.
      - Signs include hypotension, relative bradycardia:
        - ❖ Utilize vasopressors, fluid resuscitation as necessary.
    - Determine neurologic level of the injury:
      - Defined by lowest level with intact sensation and 3+/5 motor strength.
    - Assessment of degree of neurologic injury:
      - Magnitude of spinal cord involvement (**Table 13.1**).
      - American Spinal Injury Association (ASIA) impairment scale (**Table 13.2**).

**Table 13.1** Incomplete spinal cord injury manifestations

| Syndrome | Deficits | Etiology |
|---|---|---|
| Anterior cord syndrome | Paraplegia (bilateral) Pain and temperature (bilateral) Urinary retention | Injury to the anterior spinal artery |
| Central cord syndrome | Motor weakness (bilateral – arms > legs) | Hyperextension injury (i.e., syringomyelia) |
| Posterior cord syndrome | Vibration and proprioception (bilateral) | Tabes dorsalis, epidural metastases |
| Brown-Séquard | Motor (ipsilateral) Vibration and proprioception (ipsilateral) Pain and temperature 2–3 levels below lesion (contralateral) | Trauma: knife or bullet wound |

**Table 13.2** Summary of the American Spinal Injury Association (ASIA) impairment scale

| ASIA grade | Type of injury | Definition |
| --- | --- | --- |
| A | Complete | Complete loss of motor and sensory function |
| B | Incomplete | Motor function preserved below level of injury |
| C | Incomplete | Motor function preserved, but key muscles below the level of injury have a muscle grade < 3 |
| D | Incomplete | Motor function preserved, but key muscles below the level of injury have a muscle grade > 3 |
| E | Normal | No deficits |

- Standard imaging:
  - Orthogonal radiographs: anteroposterior (AP) and lateral of cervical, thoracic, and lumbar spine.
  - Computed tomography (CT) scan: sagittal and coronal reconstructions:
    - Improves visualization of occipital-cervical and cervicothoracic junctions, bony structures, and occult fractures.
  - Magnetic resonance imaging (MRI):
    - Required in cases of neurologic impairment.
    - Improves visualization of ligamentous structures.
    - Short tau inversion recovery (STIR) sequence heightens demonstration of edema.

# 13.2  Cervical Trauma and Fractures

## 13.2.1  Occipital Condyle Fracture (Fig. 13.1)

• Background and etiology:
  - Caused by high-energy trauma:
    - Axial compression or rotation.
    - Lateral bending.
    - Direct blow.

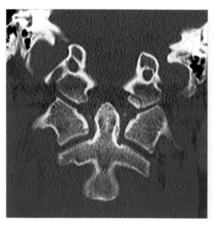

**Fig. 13.1** Coronal section. CT scan demonstrating type III occipital condyle fracture.

  - Anderson and Montesano classification system:
    ◦ Type I (15%): collapse due to axial compression; stable.
    ◦ Type II (50%): basilar skull fracture; stable.
    ◦ Type III (35%): avulsion injury near alar ligament attachment; potentially unstable.
- Presentation:
  - High cervical neck pain and stiffness.
  - Motor paresis.
  - Possible cranial nerve deficit.
- Imaging:
  - Plain radiographs: avoid traction:
    ◦ Open-mouth odontoid view.
    ◦ AP and lateral views often inadequate due to superimposition of nearby structures (maxilla, occiput, mastoid processes).
  - CT scan: cranial CT including views of the craniocervical junction.
- Management:
  - Based on presence of ligamentous injury and craniocervical stability:
    ◦ Stable: cervical orthosis.
    ◦ Unstable: occipitocervical fusion; rigid posterior segmental stabilization with instrumentation from the occiput to C2/C3.

## 13.2.2 Atlanto-Occipital Dissociation (Figs. 13.2, 13.3)

- Background and etiology:
  - Traumatic: due to high-energy, rotational or flexion–extension force causing ligamentous injury.

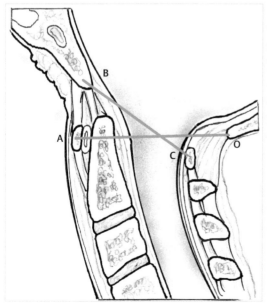

**Fig. 13.2** Lateral view. Depiction of measurements comprising the Powers ratio. A, anterior arch of C1; B, basion; C, posterior arch of C1; O, opisthion. (Reproduced with permission from Khanna AJ, ed. MRI Essentials for the Spine Specialist. New York, NY: Thieme; 2014.)

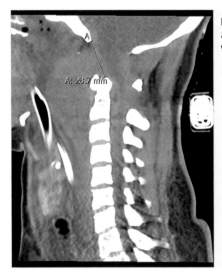

**Fig. 13.3** Sagittal section. CT scan showing a case of atlanto-occipital dissociation with a widened basion-dens interval.

- Acquired: due to bony dysplasia or ligament and soft-tissue laxity (i.e., Down's syndrome).
  - Results in separation of the spinal column from the occiput.
- Presentation:
  - Neurologic deficits and possible quadriparesis.
  - Cardiorespiratory derangement.
  - Commonly fatal due to brainstem destruction.
- Imaging:
  - Plain radiography and CT scan: lateral/sagittal views:
    - Harris' lines: suggestive of injury if:
      - Basion-dens interval (BDI) is greater than 10 mm.
      - Basion-axial interval (BAI) is greater than 12 mm.
      - Atlantodental interval (ADI) is greater than 3 mm.
      - Powers' ratio: C–D/A–B.
        - A–B: distance from anterior arch to opisthion.
        - C–D: distance from basion to posterior arch.
        - Powers' ratio greater than 1: indicative of anterior subluxation/dislocation.
        - Powers' ratio less than 1: indicative of posterior dislocation, odontoid fracture.
    - Wackenheim's line:
      - Line from the posterior surface of clivus to the upper cervical canal:
        - Line behind odontoid: posterior dissociation.
        - Line in front of odontoid: anterior dissociation.
  - MRI:
    - Used to evaluate for spinal cord and ligamentous injury.
- Management:
  - Stable: fluoroscopy-guided reduction and halo vest; avoid traction.
  - Unstable: operative posterior fusion from the occiput to at least C2.

# 13.2.3 Atlas (C1) and Jefferson's Fractures (Fig. 13.4)

- Background and etiology:
  - Due to hyperextension and axial loading causing fracture of the anterior or posterior arch of C1:
    - Combination fracture of the anterior and posterior arches is known as a **Jefferson's fracture**.
- **Presentation:**
  - Typically presents without neurologic deficits.
  - In severe fractures, possible medullary dysfunction can occur.
- Imaging:
  - Plain radiographs:
    - Open-mouth odontoid view:
      - Spence rule: greater than 7 mm composite overhang between lateral masses of C1 and C2 (39% sensitivity).
    - Lateral:
      - Atlantodental interval:
        - ❖ Less than 3 mm: normal.
        - ❖ 3–5 mm: injury to transverse ligament with intact alar and apical ligaments.
        - ❖ Greater than 5 mm: injury to transverse, alar ligament, and tectorial membrane.
  - CT scan: coronal and sagittal reconstructions:
    - Further delineate fracture pattern.
    - Aids in identifying associated injuries in the cervical spine.
    - CT angiography (CTA) to rule out vertebral artery injury.

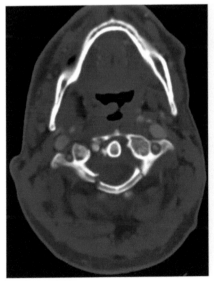

**Fig. 13.4** Axial section. CT scan showing a comminuted Jefferson fracture involving the anterior and posterior C1 arches.

- MRI:
  - ◦ Used to assess transverse of atlantal ligament (TAL).
  - ◦ Significant for possible surgical planning.
- Management: based on the patency of the TAL:
  - TAL intact: rigid cervical orthosis.
  - TAL incompetent: C1–C2 fusion.

## 13.2.4 Traumatic Spondylolisthesis of C2 (Hangman's Fracture; Fig. 13.5)

- Background and etiology:
  - Associated with high-velocity trauma.
  - Mechanistic pattern: hyperextension → compression → rebound flexion:
    - ◦ Results in bilateral fracture of the lamina and pedicles.
  - Second most common axis fracture (38%).
- Presentation:
  - Asymptomatic if nonangulated and nondisplaced.
  - Cerebellar findings (nausea, vomiting, ataxia, asymmetric neurological examination) if vertebral artery injury is present.
- Imaging:
  - Plain radiography:
    - ◦ Flexion and extension views to evaluate for subluxation.
  - Levine and Edwards radiographic classification:
    - ◦ Type I: less than 3-mm displacement.
    - ◦ Type II: greater than 3-mm displacement and greater than 11-degree angulation.
    - ◦ Type IIa: less than 3-mm displacement and greater than 11-degree angulation.
    - ◦ Type III: associated facet dislocation.

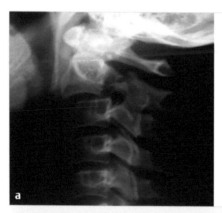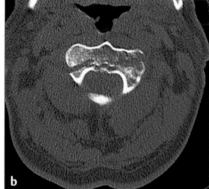

**Fig. 13.5 (a)** Lateral view. Plain radiograph demonstrating a hangman fracture at C2. **(b)** Axial section. CT scan demonstrating a comminuted hangman fracture of C2.

- CT scan with coronal and sagittal reconstructions:
  - Bilateral lamina and pedicle fracture.
  - Anterolisthesis of C2 on C3.
  - CTA to rule out vertebral artery injury.
- Management:
  - Dependent on classification:
    - Type I: halo brace for 12 weeks.
    - Type II: reduction via cervical traction and halo brace for 10 to 12 weeks.
    - Type IIa: reduction in extension followed by halo brace; avoid traction.
    - Type III: anterior C2–C3 or posterior C1–C3 fusion.

# 13.2.5 C2 Dens Fracture (Fig. 13.6)

- Background and etiology:
  - Caused by hyperflexion or hyperextension:
    - Elderly: falls.
    - Young patients: blunt trauma.
- Presentation:
  - Neck pain and tenderness to palpation.
  - Neurologic deficits usually not present.
- Imaging:
  - Radiographs: AP, lateral, and open-mouth odontoid views:
    - Anderson and D'Alonzo imaging classification:
      - Type I: avulsion fracture at the tip.
      - Type II: at the odontoid base.
      - Type III: within the C2 body.
    - Rule out os odontoideum:
      - Appears similar to a type II fracture.
      - Possible failure of fusion at base of odontoid, may be residual of an old traumatic process.
  - CT scan with sagittal and coronal reconstructions:
    - CTA required to determine vertebral artery location prior to operative therapy with posterior instrumentation.
  - MRI:
    - Used to assess integrity of the cruciate ligament.

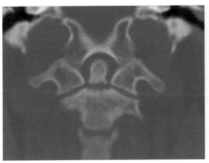

**Fig. 13.6** Coronal section. CT scan demonstrating a type II Dens fracture encompassing the base.

- Management:
  - Type 1 fractures: stable; treated with rigid cervical collar.
  - Type 2 fractures: most unstable, requires surgical treatment:
    - Anterior odontoid screw fixation.
    - Posterior C1–C2 instrumented fusion.
  - Type 3:  stable; treated with halo brace or rigid cervical collar.

## 13.2.6  Subaxial Injury Classification System (Table 13.3)

- Categorizes injury based on morphology and integrity of discoligamentous complex.
- Assigned score can guide management decisions:
  - 1–3: nonoperative therapy.
  - Greater than 5: operative therapy consisting of realignment, decompression, and stabilization.

**Table 13.3**  Subaxial injury classification

| Characteristics | Points |
| --- | --- |
| Injury morphology | |
| No abnormality | 0 |
| Compression | 1 |
| Burst | 2 |
| Distraction | 3 |
| Translation | 4 |
| Integrity of the discoligamentous complex | |
| Intact | 0 |
| Indeterminate | 1 |
| Disrupted | 2 |
| Neurological status | |
| Intact | 0 |
| Nerve root injury | 1 |
| Complete | 2 |
| Incomplete | 3 |
| Persistent cord compression | +1 |

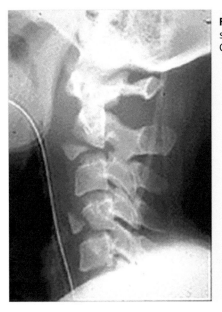

**Fig. 13.7** Lateral view. Plain radiograph showing multiple flexion teardrop fractures at C2 and C4.

## 13.2.7  Subaxial Flexion–Compression Fracture (Flexion Teardrop; Fig. 13.7)

- Background and etiology:
  - Caused by flexion–compressive forces (diving, motor vehicle collision) leading to fracture of the anteroinferior vertebral body.
- Presentation:
  - Can range from mild neurological deficits to significant radiculopathies.
  - If significant retropulsion occurs, can lead to anterior cervical cord syndrome ± quadriplegia.
- Imaging:
  - Plain radiography: lateral view:
    ◦ Fracture of the anteroinferior vertebral body ("teardrop").
    ◦ Loss of anterior vertebral body height.
    ◦ Possible displacement of posterior vertebral body into the canal.
  - CT scan:
    ◦ CTA indicated to determine possibility of blunt cerebrovascular injury.
- Management:
  - Prognosis dependent on level of spinal cord injury.
  - Stable: rigid cervical orthosis.
  - Unstable: surgical:
    ◦ Posterior fusion.
    ◦ Anterior corpectomy with strut graft and anterior cervical discectomy and fusion (ACDF).

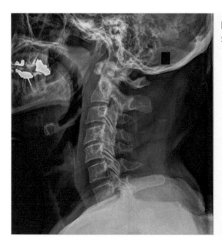

**Fig. 13.8** Lateral view. Plain radiograph showing extension teardrop fracture at C3.

## 13.2.8 Subaxial Extension–Compression Fracture (Extension Teardrop; Fig. 13.8)

- Background and etiology:
  - Caused by forced extension of the neck leading to avulsion of the anteroinferior aspect of the vertebral body via disruption of the anterior longitudinal ligament (ALL).
- Presentation:
  - Can range from mild neurological deficits to significant radiculopathies.
- Imaging:
  - Plain radiography: lateral view:
    - Anteroinferior corner fracture: usually from the ALL to the inferior corner of the vertebral body ("teardrop").
    - Widening of anterior disk space.
  - CT:
    - To determine presence of additional fractures.
    - CTA: investigation of blunt cerebrovascular injury.
- Management:
  - Typically a stable fracture: nonoperative management with rigid cervical orthosis.

## 13.2.9 Subaxial Vertical Compression (Burst) Fracture (Fig. 13.9)

- Background and etiology:
  - Caused by vertical compressive forces arising from significant trauma (i.e., diving, fall from a significant height, landing on feet).
  - Results in disruption of the anterior and posterior vertebral body cortex.
  - Often associated with posterior ligamentous injury.

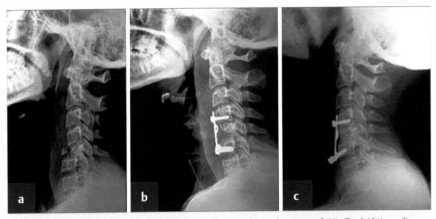

**Fig. 13.9** Lateral view. **(a)** Plain radiograph showing burst fracture of C5. **(b,c)** Plain radiograph showing corpectomy with anterior grafting and plate fixation.

- Presentation:
  - Can range from mild neurological deficits to significant radiculopathies.
  - If retropulsion occurs, can present with anterior cord syndrome.
- Imaging:
  - Plain radiography: lateral views:
    ◦ Loss of vertebral height, anterior greater than posterior.
  - CT scan:
    ◦ Burst vertebral body.
    ◦ Retropulsed fragments into the spinal canal.
  - MRI:
    ◦ Assesses for cord contusion.
- Management:
  - Stable: rigid cervical orthosis.
  - Unstable: surgical therapy:
    ◦ Corpectomy, anterior grafting, and plate fixation.

## 13.2.10  Bilateral Facet Dislocation

- Background and etiology:
  - Caused by flexion–rotation forces.
  - 10-40% percent of cases have disk herniation into the spinal canal.
- Presentation:
  - Focal neurologic deficits and radiculopathy.
- Imaging:
  - Plain radiography:
    ◦ Loss of apposition at the facet joint.
    ◦ Anterolisthesis ≥ 50%.
    ◦ Increased interspinous distance.

- MRI:
  - ○ Indications include the following:
    - Significant spinal cord deficits, paresthesias, declining mental status.
    - Following dislocation reductions.
    - Prior to operative treatment in neurologically stable patients.
- Management:
  - All patients require initial reduction:
    - ○ Awake, cooperative patient, no significant neurological deficits: reduction, followed by MRI.
    - ○ Obtunded, intoxicated patient: MRI prior to reduction to rule out disk herniation.
  - Definitive treatment requires surgical stabilization:
    - ○ ACDF ± posterior stabilization.

## 13.2.11 Unilateral Facet Dislocation (Fig. 13.10)

- Background and etiology:
  - Caused by flexion/distraction and rotation forces, leads to inferior articular facet of the superior vertebrae moving over the superior facet of the inferior vertebrae.
  - 10% of cases cause spinal cord impingement.
- Presentation:
  - Neck pain.
  - Radiculopathy (70%).
- Imaging:
  - Plain radiograph: lateral view.

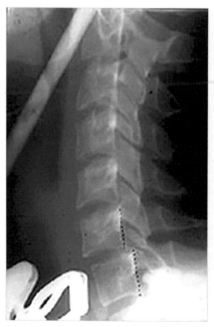

**Fig. 13.10** Lateral view. Plain radiograph showing unilateral facet dislocation with characteristic bow tie sign.

- Bow tie sign: vertebral bodies appear lateral below level of injury and oblique above level of injury.
- Anterolisthesis less than 25%.
- Interspinous widening at the affected level.
  - CT scan:
    - Useful in the detection of concomitant fractures.
  - MRI:
    - Used for detection of soft-tissue injuries, disk herniation, contusion.
- Management:
  - Stable: halo bracing for 12 weeks.
  - Unstable or presenting with radiculopathy: surgical management similar to bilateral facet dislocation:
    - ACDF ± posterior fusion.

## 13.2.12  Clay-Shoveler's Fracture

- Background and etiology:
  - Spinous process fracture caused by:
    - Stress fracture (chronic).
    - MVAs, Direct blow to posterior spine (acute).
  - Most commonly at C7 (midpoint between the lamina and spinous tip).
  - Often occurs as an isolated injury.
- Presentation:
  - Often asymptomatic.
- Imaging:
  - Plain radiography: lateral view:
    - Vertical or oblique lucency in the spinous processes:
      - Most commonly present in the lower cervical or upper thoracic areas.
    - Possible posterior displacement of fracture fragment.
- Management:
  - Stable fracture: cervical collar.

## 13.2.13   Lateral Mass Fracture (Fig. 13.11)

- Background and etiology:
  - Mechanism includes hyperextension, lateral rotation, and compression:
    - Motor vehicle accident, falls, objects falling on head.
  - Ipsilateral fracture of the pedicle and lamina.
  - Affects two adjacent motion segments due to involvement of the facet joints.
- Presentation:
  - High degree of instability leading to neurological deficits (66%).
- Imaging:
  - Plain radiography:
    - Poor sensitivity: 38%.
    - Disk space narrowing and instability.

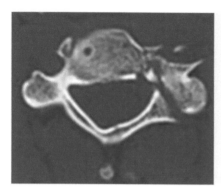

**Fig. 13.11** Axial section. CT scan showing a cervical lateral mass fracture involving the pedicle and lamina.

- CT:
  - Translation of fractured and adjacent vertebrae in multiple planes.
  - Vertebral body destruction.
  - Used for evaluation of translation of fractured vertebrae.
- MRI:
  - Disruption of ligaments:
    - ALL: 50 to 75%.
    - PLL: 30 to 35%.
    - Interspinous and supraspinous ligaments: 10 to 75%.
- Management:
  - Stable injuries without neurologic deficits: halo vest.
  - Most cases are unstable: require surgical treatment:
    - Posterior decompression with two-level instrumented fusion.

# 13.3  Thoracolumbar Fractures

## 13.3.1  General Background

- The most common location is the T11–L2 region:
  - Susceptible to injury due to transition from fixed, kyphotic thoracic spine → mobile, lordotic lumbar spine.
- Operative indications include the following:
  - Instability due to posterior ligamentous injury.
  - Focal neurologic deficits or progressive decrease in neurologic status.

## 13.3.2  Thoracolumbar Injury Classification System (Table 13.4)

- Categorizes injuries based on injury morphology, neurologic injury, posterior ligamentous complex integrity.
- Management recommendations are based on total score:
  - 3 or lower: nonoperative treatment.
  - 4: indeterminate.
  - 5 or higher: operative intervention.

**Table 13.4** Injury classification system for thoracolumbar spine

| Component | Qualifiers | Score |
|---|---|---|
| Morphology type | | |
| Compression | | 1 |
| Burst | | 1 |
| Translational/rotational | | 3 |
| Distraction | | 4 |
| Neurological involvement | | |
| Intact | | 0 |
| Nerve root | | 2 |
| Cord, conus medullaris | Complete | 2 |
| | Incomplete | 3 |
| Cauda equina | | 3 |
| Posterior ligamentous complex | | |
| Intact | | 0 |
| Injury suspected/indeterminate | | 2 |
| Injured | | 3 |

## 13.3.3 Compressive Thoracolumbar Fracture (Fig. 13.12)

• Background and etiology:
  - Most common fragility fracture, often secondary to osteoporosis; often a result of a fall.
• Presentation:
  - Localized pain (25%).
  - Mortality increases with concomitant hip fracture.
  - Important to rule out metastatic disease (atypical radiograph, failure to thrive, fracture in a young patient without trauma, fractures above T5 level).
• Imaging:
  - Plain radiographs:
    ○ Loss of vertebral height of at least 20%.
    ○ Unstable fractures are those with greater than 50% loss of vertebral height, greater than 30 degree angulation, greater than 30 degree focal kyphosis.
  - CT and MRI generally not necessary for diagnosis:
    ○ MRI can be used to identify chronicity of injury, assess for spinal cord compression, edema, or hemorrhage.
• Management:
  - Full medical workup.
  - Stable fractures: thoracolumbosacral orthosis (TLSO) or Lewitt extension bracing.
  - Unstable fractures with pain or loss of mobility: vertebroplasty or kyphoplasty.

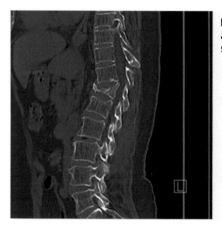

**Fig. 13.12** Sagittal section. CT scan showing a compression fracture of the thoracolumbar spine.

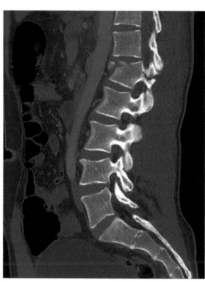

**Fig. 13.13** Lateral view. Radiograph showing a chance fracture with significant anterior wedging.

### 13.3.4  Chance Fracture ("Seatbelt Fracture"; Fig. 13.13)

- Background and etiology:
  - Flexion–distraction mechanism; often occurs in motor vehicle accidents in backseat passengers wearing a seatbelt.
  - Fracture traversing all three columns of the vertebrae.
  - Can be isolated bony or ligamentous injury.
- Presentation:
  - Associated with a high rate of gastrointestinal injury (50% of cases present with concomitant perforated viscus).

- Imaging:
  - Radiography: lateral view:
    - Anterior wedge fracture of the vertebral body.
    - Horizontal fracture through posterior elements or distraction of spinous processes and facet joints.
  - CT:
    - Used to evaluate for retropulsion of bony fragments into the spinal canal.
  - MRI:
    - Used to evaluate posterior elements.
- Management:
  - Stable fracture without ligamentous injury: TLSO body brace or cast.
  - Unstable fracture with ligamentous injury: posterior spinal fusion.

# 13.3.5 Thoracolumbar Burst Fracture (Fig. 13.14)

- Background and etiology:
  - Caused by axial loading, resulting in disruption of the posterior vertebral body cortex.
  - Most commonly occurs at the thoracolumbar junction.
- Presentation:
  - Canal compromise leads to initial neurologic dysfunction and possible anterior cord syndrome.
  - Other spinal fractures also occur in 20% of cases.
- Imaging:
  - Plain radiographs: AP and lateral views:
    - Widening of interpedicular space.
    - Vertebral collapse.
    - Kyphosis.
    - Possible retropulsed fragments.
  - CT:
    - Required if neurologic deficit present in lower extremity.

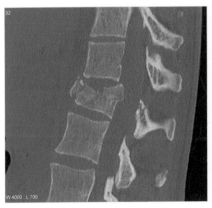

**Fig. 13.14** Sagittal section. CT scan showing a thoracolumbar burst fracture with retropulsion.

- MRI:
  - Spinal cord compression, contusion, edema, hemorrhage.
  - Posterior ligamentous complex injury.
- Management:
  - Stable fractures: less than 50% vertebral collapse, less than 30 degree kyphosis, less than 50% lumbar canal collapse, neurologically intact:
    - Thoracolumbar orthosis.
  - Unstable fractures: surgical decompression with spine stabilization:
    - Combined anterior and posterior approach.

# 13.4  Sacral Fracture (Fig. 13.15)

- Background and etiology:
  - Occurs after a fall from a height (elderly) or during high-energy trauma.
  - Often appears along with pelvic injuries (30–45%).
- Presentation:
  - Peripelvic pain.
  - Neurologic deficits based on location.
  - If sacral roots are involved: bowel and bladder dysfunction.
  - Denis' classification:
    - Zone 1: fracture lateral to the sacral foramina:
      - Most common type of sacral fracture.
      - Less than 10% with neurologic injury, affects L5.
    - Zone 2: through sacral foramina:
      - Causes unilateral neurologic deficits.
    - Zone 3: through the body, medial to the sacral foramina:
      - Most commonly presents with neurologic deficits (56%).
- Imaging:
  - Radiographic views: AP, inlet, outlet, lateral:
    - Multiple views required as these fractures are commonly missed (only 30% shown on radiographs).
  - CT reconstruction: gold standard:
    - Coronal and sagittal reconstructions.

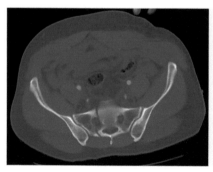

**Fig. 13.15** Axial section. CT scan showing a zone II fracture of the sacrum.

- MRI: recommended when neurologic deficits are present or compromise is expected.
- Management:
  - Prognosis and outcome directly related to the presence of neurologic injury.
  - Stable fractures: less than 1 cm displacement, no neurologic deficits:
    ◦ Nonoperative therapy: progressive weight bearing and orthosis.
  - Unstable fractures: greater than 1 cm displacement, persistent pain, soft-tissue involvement:
    ◦ Surgical reduction and fixation.
    ◦ Iliopelvic reconstruction may be required to allow for adequate weight bearing.

# Suggested Readings

1. Al-Mahfoudh R, Beagrie C, Woolley E, et al. Management of typical and atypical hangman's fractures. Global Spine J 2016;6(3):248–256
2. Atlas SW, Regenbogen V, Rogers LF, Kim KS. The radiographic characterization of burst fractures of the spine. AJR Am J Roentgenol 1986;147(3):575–582
3. Bernstein MP, Mirvis SE, Shanmuganathan K. Chance-type fractures of the thoracolumbar spine: imaging analysis in 53 patients. AJR Am J Roentgenol 2006;187(4):859–868
4. Davis JM, Beall DP, Lastine C, Sweet C, Wolff J, Wu D. Chance fracture of the upper thoracic spine. AJR Am J Roentgenol 2004;183(5):1475–1478
5. Denis F, Davis S, Comfort T. Sacral fractures: an important problem. Retrospective analysis of 236 cases. Clin Orthop Relat Res 1988;227(227):67–81
6. Giauque AP, Bittle MM, Braman JP. Type I hangman's fracture. Curr Probl Diagn Radiol 2012;41(4):116–117
7. Hak DJ, Baran S, Stahel P. Sacral fractures: current strategies in diagnosis and management. Orthopedics 2009;32(10):752–757
8. Kasliwal MK, Fontes RB, Traynelis VC. Occipitocervical dissociation-incidence, evaluation, and treatment. Curr Rev Musculoskelet Med 2016;9(3):247–254
9. Kim KS, Chen HH, Russell EJ, Rogers LF. Flexion teardrop fracture of the cervical spine: radiographic characteristics. AJR Am J Roentgenol 1989;152(2):319–326
10. Kirshblum SC, Biering-Sørensen F, Betz R, et al. International standards for neurological classification of spinal cord injury: cases with classification challenges. Top Spinal Cord Inj Rehabil 2014;20(2):81–89
11. Kondo KL. Osteoporotic vertebral compression fractures and vertebral augmentation. Semin Intervent Radiol 2008;25(4):413–424
12. Lee P, Hunter TB, Taljanovic M. Musculoskeletal colloquialisms: how did we come up with these names? Radiographics 2004;24(4):1009–1027
13. Lenchik L, Rogers LF, Delmas PD, Genant HK. Diagnosis of osteoporotic vertebral fractures: importance of recognition and description by radiologists. AJR Am J Roentgenol 2004;183(4):949–958
14. Leone A, Cerase A, Colosimo C, Lauro L, Puca A, Marano P. Occipital condylar fractures: a review. Radiology 2000;216(3):635–644
15. Noble ER, Smoker WR. The forgotten condyle: the appearance, morphology, and classification of occipital condyle fractures. AJNR Am J Neuroradiol 1996;17(3):507–513

16. O'Shaughnessy J, Grenier JM, Stern PJ. A delayed diagnosis of bilateral facet dislocation of the cervical spine: a case report. J Can Chiropr Assoc 2014;58(1):45–51

17. Rao SK, Wasyliw C, Nunez DB Jr. Spectrum of imaging findings in hyperextension injuries of the neck. Radiographics 2005;25(5):1239–1254

18. Riascos R, Bonfante E, Cotes C, Guirguis M, Hakimelahi R, West C. Imaging of atlanto-occipital and atlantoaxial traumatic injuries: what the radiologist needs to know. Radiographics 2015;35(7):2121–2134

19. Rojas CA, Bertozzi JC, Martinez CR, Whitlow J. Reassessment of the craniocervical junction: normal values on CT. AJNR Am J Neuroradiol 2007;28(9):1819–1823

20. Shapiro SA. Management of unilateral locked facet of the cervical spine. Neurosurgery 1993;33(5):832–837, discussion 837

21. Shuman WP, Rogers JV, Sickler ME, et al. Thoracolumbar burst fractures: CT dimensions of the spinal canal relative to postsurgical improvement. AJR Am J Roentgenol 1985;145(2):337–341

22. Solaroğlu I, Kaptanoğlu E, Okutan O, Beşkonakli E. Multiple isolated spinous process fracture (Clay-shoveler's fracture) of cervical spine: a case report. Ulus Travma Acil Cerrahi Derg 2007;13(2):162–164

23. Koh YD, Kim DJ, Koh YW. Reliability and validity of Thoracolumbar Injury Classification and Severity Score (TLICS). Asian Spine J 2010;4(2):109–117

24. Kotani Y, Abumi K, Ito M, Minami A. Cervical spine injuries associated with lateral mass and facet joint fractures: new classification and surgical treatment with pedicle screw fixation. Eur Spine J 2005;14(1):69–77

25. Lee SH, Sung JK. Unilateral lateral mass-facet fractures with rotational instability: new classification and a review of 39 cases treated conservatively and with single segment anterior fusion. J Trauma 2009;66(3):758–767

26. Vaccaro AR, Hulbert RJ, Patel AA, et al; Spine Trauma Study Group. The subaxial cervical spine injury classification system: a novel approach to recognize the importance of morphology, neurology, and integrity of the disco-ligamentous complex. Spine 2007;32(21):2365–2374

# 14 Primary and Metastatic Spinal Tumors

*Ankur S. Narain, Fady Y. Hijji, Philip K. Louie, Daniel D. Bohl, and Kern Singh*

## 14.1 Introduction

Primary and metastatic spinal neoplasms represent a series of complex pathologies that range from benign to life threatening. Detection of spinal neoplasms is further hindered by their indolent progression and vague symptomatology. As such, it is important for the practitioner to understand the nuances in examination and radiographic findings that are present in these patients. Furthermore, as these cases are often complex, understanding of the appropriate timing of nonoperative versus operative management is necessary to ensure the best possible clinical outcome.

## 14.2 Background and Etiology

- Metastatic spinal lesions are much more common than primary lesions.
- 10-30% of new cancer diagnoses have spinal metastases at discovery:
  - Spine is the most common site of metastatic bone disease.
- Affects thoracic spine (68–70%) > lumbosacral spine (16–22%) > cervical spine (8–15%).

## 14.3 Presentation and Physical Examination Findings (Table 14.1)

- Most common clinical presentation is axial back pain (85–96%).
- Progressive, nonmechanical, nighttime pain.
- Neurological symptoms: radiculopathy or myelopathy:
  - Changes in fine motor skills.
  - Gait and balance instability.

**Table 14.1** Classic physical examination findings in metastatic spine tumors

| Primary tumors | Physical examination findings |
| --- | --- |
| Breast | Fixed, hard, nontender breast mass<br>Nipple retraction |
| Prostate cancer | Nodularity in the prostate on digital rectal examination |
| Thyroid cancer | Painless, palpable thyroid |
| Lung cancer | Cough, hemoptysis |
| Renal cell carcinoma | Hematuria, flank pain, abdominal mass |

– Bowel and bladder dysfunction.
– Pathologic reflexes.
• Pathologic fractures with subsequent kyphosis.
• Weight loss.

# 14.4 Imaging

• Plain radiography:
  – Odontoid, swimmer's, and upright views of the entire spine.
  – Assesses spinal alignment, stability, presence of metastatic lesions, and presence of compression fractures.
  – Identifies osteolytic and osteoblastic lesions:
    ○ Osteolytic: areas of severe bone loss due to excess osteoclast activity, appears as area of radiolucency.
    ○ Osteoblastic: areas of excess bone formation due to osteoblast activity, appears as areas of radiodensity.
  – "Winking owl" sign: lysis of pedicular cortical bone (high sensitivity).
  – Osseous lesions often not visible on plain radiographs until destruction of greater than 50% of the vertebral body has occurred.
• Computed tomography (CT):
  – Useful for surgical planning and visualization of bone destruction.
  – Myelography to evaluate for impingement.
  – Imaging of the chest, abdomen, and pelvis is required for staging.
  – Poor overall sensitivity (66%).
• Magnetic resonance imaging (MRI) ± gadolinium contrast:
  – T1, T2, and short tau inversion recovery (STIR) weighted images (98.7% sensitivity).
  – Pedicular involvement, edematous regions with defined borders, noncontiguous involvement are common findings.
  – Contrast aids in the evaluation of soft tissue, epidural space, and spinal cord.
• Bone scintigraphy: technetium-99m:
  – Shows increased uptake in regions of neoplastic involvement.
  – Low sensitivity for differentiating metastatic disease from osteoporotic compression fractures, infection, or degenerative changes.

# 14.5 Diagnosis and Staging

• CT-guided biopsy:
  – Gold standard for tissue analysis:
    ○ 76% sensitivity for sclerotic lesions; 93% sensitivity for lytic lesions.
  – Percutaneous approach preferred; open approach may be utilized when percutaneous biopsy is negative but concern for tumor burden remains high.
  – If the lesion is metastatic, biopsy of primary disease site is preferred.
• Staging:
  – Weinstein–Boriani–Biagini system (**Fig. 14.1**):

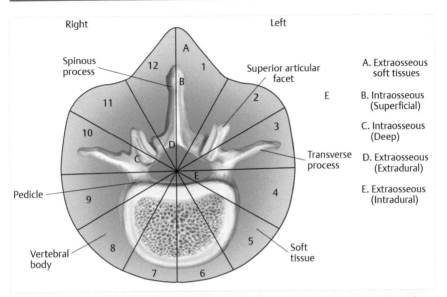

**Fig. 14.1** Weinstein–Boriani–Biagini staging system for spinal neoplasms. (Reproduced with permission from An HS, Singh K, eds. Synopsis of Spine Surgery. 3rd edition. New York, NY: Thieme; 2016).

- ○ Three-dimensional description of tumor invasion:
  - ▪ Twelve pielike zones rotating in a clockwise fashion starting at the spinous process.
  - ▪ Notes involvement of different vertebral layers: extraosseous soft tissue (A), superficial intraosseous (B), deep intraosseous (C), extradural extraosseous (D), intradural extraosseous (E).
  - ▪ Specifies the involved spinal segment.

# 14.6 Primary Spinal Tumors (Figs. 14.2, 14.3, Tables 14.2–14.5)

## 14.6.1 Metastatic Spinal Tumors (Fig. 14.4)

- Background and etiology:
  - Highest incidence between ages of 40 and 60 years.
  - Affects males more often than females.
  - Most common metastatic primary neoplasms:
    - ○ Breast cancer.
    - ○ Lung cancer.
    - ○ Thyroid cancer.
    - ○ Prostate cancer.
    - ○ Renal cell carcinoma (RCC).
  - Can spread via primary neoplasms by hematogenous, direct, or cerebrospinal fluid (CSF) extension:

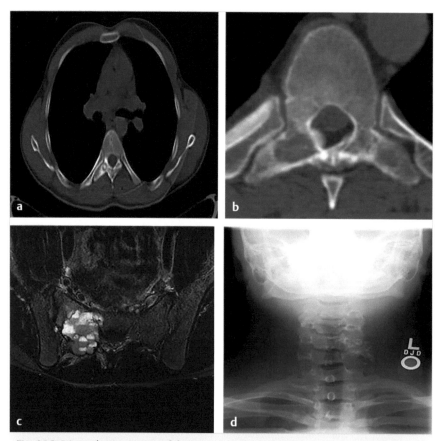

**Fig. 14.2** Primary benign tumors of the spine. **(a)** Axial section. CT scan showing osteoid osteoma of the thoracic spine. Note the lesion in the right-sided posterior elements. **(b)** Axial section. CT scan showing osteoblastoma of the thoracic spine. Note the lesion in the right-sided posterior elements. **(c)** Axial section. CT scan showing a giant cell tumor of the right-sided sacrum. **(d)** Anteroposterior view. Radiograph depicting an osteochondroma at the left-sided C5–C6 levels. (Reproduced with permission from An HS, Singh K, eds. Synopsis of Spine Surgery. 3rd ed. New York, NY: Thieme; 2016.)

- ◦ Hematogenous extension can affect multiple levels via Baton's venous plexus.
  - ◦ Most mechanistic evidence points toward tumor cell disassociation from a primary mass, penetration of the surrounding extracellular matrix, travel through lymphatic or blood vessels, and seeding of a distant site.
  - – Lesions often located in one of three compartments:
    - ◦ Extradural: most common.
    - ◦ Intradural–extramedullary.
    - ◦ Intramedullary.
- • Presentation:
  - – Similar to primary neoplasms:
    - ◦ Pain (83–95%).
    - ◦ Constitutional symptoms.

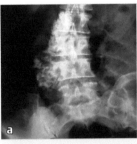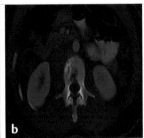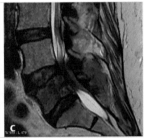

**Fig. 14.3** Primary malignant tumors of the spine. **(a)** Anteroposterior view. Radiograph showing a large chondrosarcoma of the transverse processes of the lumbar spine. **(b)** Axial section. CT scan showing Ewing's sarcoma of L2. Note the mixed lytic and blastic lesions present in the right lateral aspect of the vertebral body. **(c)** Sagittal section. T2-weighted MRI showing primary lymphoma affecting L5, leading to complete replacement of normal bone marrow and compression of the cauda equina.

**Table 14.2** Benign neoplasms of the spine

| Tumor | Age | Gender | Location | Radiographic findings | Symptoms | Treatment |
|---|---|---|---|---|---|---|
| Osteoid osteoma | < 30 y | M > F | Posterior elements | Sclerosis surrounding a radiolucent nidus (15- to 20-mm diameter) | Back pain Pain relieved by anti-inflammatories (salicylates, NSAIDs, COX-2 inhibitors) | Anti-inflammatories En bloc resection if fixed spinal deformity |
| Osteoblastoma | < 30 y | M > F | Posterior elements Lumbar spine predominant | Similar to osteoid osteoma Radiolucent nidus > 20 mm diameter | Dull back pain ±Neural compression | En bloc resection ± Fusion if instability present |
| Aneurysmal bone cyst | < 20 y | F > M | Posterior elements 70% in thoracolumbar region | Axial deformity | Slowly progressive pain Palpable mass Possible deformity | En bloc resection ± stabilization if instability present |
| Osteochondroma | > 30 y | M > F | Posterior elements Primarily cervical region | Deformity Mature cortical and medullary bone continual with underlying bone | Pain and swelling in affected areas | En bloc resection ± stabilization |
| Giant cell tumor | 20–50 y | F > M | Vertebral body | Expansile, lytic lesion with sclerotic rim Compression fractures | Back pain ± radiating pain Spinal cord compression | En bloc resection ± Adjuvant therapy if resection not viable |

*(Continued)*

**Table 14.2** (*Continued*)

| Tumor | Age | Gender | Location | Radiographic findings | Symptoms | Treatment |
|---|---|---|---|---|---|---|
| Eosinophilic granuloma | < 10 y | M > F | Vertebral body Thoracic region | Lytic lesions in vertebral body Vertebra plana | Persistent back pain Restricted ROM Deformity Diabetes insipidus (pituitary involvement) | Rest ± analgesics as necessary |
| Hemangioma | Variable | M=F | Thoracic and lumbar spine | Corduroy patterns with vertical striations | Often asymptomatic Possible pain, neurodeficits | Only if symptomatic Radiation therapy Transarterial embolization Vertebroplasty/ kyphoplasty |

Abbreviations: COX-2, cyclooxygenase-2; NSAIDs, nonsteroidal anti-inflammatory drugs; ROM, range of motion.

**Table 14.3**  Primary malignant tumors of the spine

| Tumor | Age | Gender | Location | Radiographic findings | Symptoms | Treatment |
|---|---|---|---|---|---|---|
| Solitary plasmacytoma | > 50 y | M > F | Vertebral body | Punched-out lytic lesions | Spinal cord compression Pathologic fractures Possible paraparesis | Radiotherapy ± surgical stabilization Follow response to treatment via M light chain levels on serum protein electrophoresis |
| Chordoma | < 40 y | M > F | Sacrum, C1–C2 | T2-weighted MRI is the modality of choice High T2 signal intensity, soft-tissue tumor extension | Nonspecific low back pain Rectal dysfunction Radiculopathy | En bloc resection with clear margins Must warn patients of possible bladder, bowel, and sexual dysfunction |
| Primary lymphoma | 40–60 y | M > F | Vertebral body | Osteolytic lesions Ivory vertebrae | Local pain Spinal cord compression | Decompression via laminectomy + systemic chemo- and radiotherapy |

(Continued)

**Table 14.3** (Continued)

| Tumor | Age | Gender | Location | Radiographic findings | Symptoms | Treatment |
|---|---|---|---|---|---|---|
| Chondro-sarcoma | > 40 y | M > F | Vertebral body | Bony destruction Soft-tissue mass with matrix calcification | Pain Neurologic deficit | En bloc surgical resection |
| Osteosar-coma | < 20 y | M > F | Vertebral body | Mixed lytic and sclerotic lesions with cortical destruction | Pain Neurologic deficit due to cord compression | En bloc local excision Radiation and chemotheapy |
| Ewing's sarcoma | < 20 y | M > F | Vertebral body | Mottled, moth-eaten appearance Irregular bone destruction with ill-defined margins Soft-tissue mass | Pain, swelling Systemic symptoms (fever) Neurologic deficits due to cord compression | Combined radiation and chemotherapy Surgery reserved for cases with instability and neurologic deficit |

Abbreviation: MRI, magnetic resonance imaging.

**Table 14.4** Intraspinal neoplasms or cysts

| Tumor | Age | Gender | Radiographic findings | Treatment | Symptoms | Notes |
|---|---|---|---|---|---|---|
| Schwanno-ma | 20-50 y | M = F | Circular filling defect on myelogram | Surgical excision | Shooting pain and paresthesias upon nerve palpation | Most common spinal nerve or cord tumor Common in patients with neurofibromatosis (67%) |
| Meningi-oma | 40–50 y | F > M | Solid, well-circumscribed lesion with broad dural attachment | Surgical excision | Pain, not reproducible on palpation | Primarily solitary lesions (90%) Involve multiple nerve fascicles and travel parallel to the nerve |
| Neurofibro-ma | 20–30 y | - | Dumb-bell-shaped, circular defect Vertebral erosion and rib thinning | Surgical excision Adjuvant therapy if resection is incomplete | Pain ± weakness, possible paralysis Possible deformity | 80–90% of spinal involvement is in the thoracic region More commonly intracranial |

**Table 14.5** Intradural intramedullary tumors

| Tumor | Age | Gender | Radiographic findings | Treatment | Symptoms | Notes |
|---|---|---|---|---|---|---|
| Astrocytoma | 40–60 y | M > F | Expansile lesions with ill-defined borders Spans multiple vertebral segments | Surgical excision | Pain Sensory deficits Motor deficits distal to the spinal levels of involvement | Arise from glial cell transformation |
| Ependymoma | 30–40 y | M = F | Areas of cystic change with cord expansion High-signal intensity intraparenchymally | Surgical excision | Back pain Paresthesia Sensory loss Lower extremity spasticity | Arise from cuboidal ependymal cells Most common adult primary spinal parenchymal neoplasm |

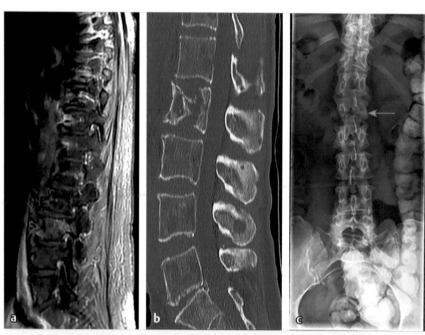

**Fig. 14.4** Metastatic tumors of the spine. **(a)** Sagittal view. T1-weighted MRI showing multiple lytic metastatic lesions derived from renal cell carcinoma. **(b)** Sagittal section. CT scan showing multiple lytic lesions arising from breast cancer. Note the presence of a pathologic fracture in the L2 vertebral body. **(c)** Anteroposterior view. Radiograph showing the classic winking owl sign at L2 (*arrow*), associated with lytic activity within pedicular bone. This sign is often associated with metastatic spinal lesions.

- Motor, autonomic dysfunction due to metastatic spinal cord compression.
- Sensory and motor dysfunction.
- Imaging:
  - Plain radiographs:
    - Osteolytic lesions in the majority of cases.
    - Osteoblastic lesions if primary lesion is prostate or breast cancer.
    - Pathologic and compression fractures.
    - Deformity.
  - Bone scan:
    - Can reveal other metastatic lesions at an earlier stage than plain radiography.
  - CT scan:
    - Improved visualization of bony anatomy.
    - Important for determination of primary neoplasm and other areas of metastasis.
  - MRI:
    - Gold standard: allows for superior resolution of soft tissue, disk space, spinal cord, and nerve roots.
    - The degree of cord compression has been objectified via the metastatic epidural spinal cord compression scale:
      - Grade 0: bone disease only.
      - Grade 1a: epidural impingement without thecal sac deformation.
      - Grade 1b: deformation of the thecal sac without spinal cord abutment.
      - Grade 1c: deformation of the thecal sac and spinal cord abutment, but without cord compression.
      - Grade 2: spinal cord compression with visible CSF around the cord.
      - Grade 3: spinal cord compression with no visible CSF around the cord.
  - Angiography:
    - Required when primary tumors are highly vascular (thyroid, RCC).
    - Allows for surgical planning and possible preoperative embolization to control hemorrhage.

## 14.6.2 Management (Table 14.6)

- Decision framework for treatment of metastatic spine disease:
  - The Neurologic, Oncologic, Mechanical Instability, and Systemic Disease (NOMS) framework: approach to the treatment of spinal metastatic tumors.
  - Provides a framework via four functional assessments: neurologic, oncologic, mechanical, and systemic diseases.
- Symptomatic therapy:
  - Analgesia.
  - Corticosteroids:
    - Reduce pain via decreasing tumor inflammation and edema.
  - Bisphosphonates:
    - Reduces the risk of pathologic fracture, pain due to lytic lesions.
    - Lowers hypercalcemia of malignancy.

**Table 14.6** The NOMS framework for treatment of metastatic spine disease

| Neurologic |
| --- |
| Radiographic evidence of epidural spinal cord compression |
| Clinical assessment of myelopathy |
| Clinical assessment of functional radiculopathy |

| Oncologic |
| --- |
| Expected response to treatment |
| Durability of response to various treatments, including: SRS, EBRT, immunotherapy, biologics, chemotherapy, hormone treatment |

| Mechanical instability |
| --- |
| Associated with pathologic fractures |
| Treatment options include: brace, percutaneous cement, and/or pedicle screw augmentation, open surgery |

| Systemic disease |
| --- |
| Presence of medical comorbidities |
| Ability to tolerate proposed treatment modalities |
| Overall expected survival based on disease severity and tumor histological factors |

Abbreviations: EBRT, external beam radiation therapy; NOMS, Neurologic, Oncologic, Mechanical Instability, and Systemic Disease; SRS, stereotactic radiosurgery.

- Radiation therapy:
  - Mainstay of therapy.
  - Indications include the following:
    - Radiosensitive tumors (hematopoietic, prostate, breast) without spinal instability.
    - Diffuse spinal involvement.
    - Contraindication or inability to tolerate surgery.
- Targeted medical treatments:
  - Efficacy varies with oncologic diagnosis.
  - Combinations of tyrosine kinase inhibitors, monoclonal antibodies, and other targeted immunotherapy drugs have shown improved outcomes compared to traditional cytotoxic chemotherapy.
- Preoperative embolization:
  - Necessary for hypervascular metastatic lesions:
    - An accurate mapping of the arterial geography is crucial.
    - Often performed within 48 hours of the planned procedure.
- Hormonal therapy:
  - Used for metastatic spinal lesions:
    - Prostate cancer: gonadotropin-releasing hormone (GnRH) agonists ± flutamide.
    - Breast cancer: estrogen antagonists and aromatase inhibitors.
- Stereotactic radiosurgery:
  - Delivers high doses of radiation to small foci of tissue.
  - Novel approach that allows for greater lesion targeting and minimization of radiation exposure to normal tissues.
  - Can be administered in an outpatient setting.

• Surgical therapy with adjuvant radiotherapy:
  - Indications include the following:
    ◦ Tumors resistant to radiation therapy or a previously failed radiation therapy course.
    ◦ Curative excision.
    ◦ Rapid neurological decline or epidural cord compression.
    ◦ Anatomic instability.
    ◦ Necessity of tissue diagnosis.
    ◦ Intractable pain.
  - Approach can be anterior or posterior depending on the tumor location:
    ◦ Anterior approach: vertebral body involvement.
    ◦ Posterior approach: used if instrumented stabilization is needed.
  - Vertebroplasty or kyphoplasty can also be used for the treatment of pain, pathologic fractures:
    ◦ Kyphoplasty may also improve spinal kyphosis due to balloon expansion.

## Suggested Readings

1.  Brihaye J, Ectors P, Lemort M, Van Houtte P. The management of spinal epidural metastases. Adv Tech Stand Neurosurg 1988;16:121–176
2.  Buhmann Kirchhoff S, Becker C, Duerr HR, Reiser M, Baur-Melnyk A. Detection of osseous metastases of the spine: comparison of high resolution multi-detector-CT with MRI. Eur J Radiol 2009;69(3):567–573
3.  Gilbert RW, Kim JH, Posner JB. Epidural spinal cord compression from metastatic tumor: diagnosis and treatment. Ann Neurol 1978;3(1):40–51
4.  Lis E, Bilsky MH, Pisinski L, et al. Percutaneous CT-guided biopsy of osseous lesion of the spine in patients with known or suspected malignancy. AJNR Am J Neuroradiol 2004;25(9):1583–1588
5.  Mesfin A, Buchowski JM, Gokaslan ZL, Bird JE. Management of metastatic cervical spine tumors. J Am Acad Orthop Surg 2015;23(1):38–46
6.  Rose PS, Buchowski JM. Metastatic disease in the thoracic and lumbar spine: evaluation and management. J Am Acad Orthop Surg 2011;19(1):37–48
7.  Schiff D, O'Neill BP, Suman VJ. Spinal epidural metastasis as the initial manifestation of malignancy: clinical features and diagnostic approach. Neurology 1997;49(2):452–456
8.  Tatsui H, Onomura T, Morishita S, Oketa M, Inoue T. Survival rates of patients with metastatic spinal cancer after scintigraphic detection of abnormal radioactive accumulation. Spine 1996;21(18):2143–2148
9.  Thakur NA, Daniels AH, Schiller J, et al. Benign tumors of the spine. J Am Acad Orthop Surg 2012;20(11):715–724
10. White AP, Kwon BK, Lindskog DM, Friedlaender GE, Grauer JN. Metastatic disease of the spine. J Am Acad Orthop Surg 2006;14(11):587–598
11. Bertram C, Madert J, Eggers C. Eosinophilic granuloma of the cervical spine. Spine 2002;27(13):1408–1413
12. Currier BL, Papagelopoulos PJ, Krauss WE, Unni KK, Yaszemski MJ. Total en bloc spondylectomy of C5 vertebra for chordoma. Spine 2007;32(9):E294–E299

13. Dimopoulos MA, Goldstein J, Fuller L, Delasalle K, Alexanian R. Curability of solitary bone plasmacytoma. J Clin Oncol 1992;10(4):587–590
14. Fourney DR, Rhines LD, Hentschel SJ, et al. En bloc resection of primary sacral tumors: classification of surgical approaches and outcome. J Neurosurg Spine 2005;3(2):111–122
15. Fuchs B, Dickey ID, Yaszemski MJ, Inwards CY, Sim FH. Operative management of sacral chordoma. J Bone Joint Surg Am 2005;87(10):2211–2216
16. Garg S, Mehta S, Dormans JP. Langerhans cell histiocytosis of the spine in children. Long-term follow-up. J Bone Joint Surg Am 2004;86-A(8):1740–1750
17. Hay MC, Paterson D, Taylor TK. Aneurysmal bone cysts of the spine. J Bone Joint Surg Br 1978;60-B(3):406–411
18. Huang W, Yang X, Cao D, et al. Eosinophilic granuloma of spine in adults: a report of 30 cases and outcome. Acta Neurochir (Wien) 2010;152(7):1129–1137
19. Hulen CA, Temple HT, Fox WP, Sama AA, Green BA, Eismont FJ. Oncologic and functional outcome following sacrectomy for sacral chordoma. J Bone Joint Surg Am 2006;88(7):1532–1539
20. Jackson RP, Reckling FW, Mants FA. Osteoid osteoma and osteoblastoma. Similar histologic lesions with different natural histories. Clin Orthop Relat Res 1977; (128):303–313
21. Kawahara N, Tomita K, Fujita T, Maruo S, Otsuka S, Kinoshita G. Osteosarcoma of the thoracolumbar spine: total en bloc spondylectomy. A case report. J Bone Joint Surg Am 1997;79(3):453–458
22. Knowling MA, Harwood AR, Bergsagel DE. Comparison of extramedullary plasmacytomas with solitary and multiple plasma cell tumors of bone. J Clin Oncol 1983;1(4):255–262
23. Liebross RH, Ha CS, Cox JD, Weber D, Delasalle K, Alexanian R. Solitary bone plasmacytoma: outcome and prognostic factors following radiotherapy. Int J Radiat Oncol Biol Phys 1998;41(5):1063–1067
24. Nilsson PM, Kandell-Collén A, Andersson HI. Blood pressure and metabolic factors in relation to chronic pain. Blood Press 1997;6(5):294–298
25. Sanjay BK, Sim FH, Unni KK, McLeod RA, Klassen RA. Giant-cell tumours of the spine. J Bone Joint Surg Br 1993;75(1):148–154
26. Swee RG, McLeod RA, Beabout JW. Osteoid osteoma. Detection, diagnosis, and localization. Radiology 1979;130(1):117–123
27. Wuisman P, Lieshout O, Sugihara S, van Dijk M. Total sacrectomy and reconstruction: oncologic and functional outcome. Clin Orthop Relat Res 2000;(381):192–203
28. Yeom JS, Lee CK, Shin HY, Lee CS, Han CS, Chang H. Langerhans' cell histiocytosis of the spine. Analysis of twenty-three cases. Spine 1999;24(16):1740–1749
29. York JE, Kaczaraj A, Abi-Said D, et al. Sacral chordoma: 40-year experience at a major cancer center. Neurosurgery 1999;44(1):74–79, discussion 79–80
30. Abd-El-Barr MM, Huang KT, Chi JH. Infiltrating spinal cord astrocytomas: epidemiology, diagnosis, treatments and future directions. J Clin Neurosci 2016;29:15–20
31. Abul-Kasim K, Thurnher MM, McKeever P, Sundgren PC. Intradural spinal tumors: current classification and MRI features. Neuroradiology 2008;50(4):301–314
32. Celano E, Salehani A, Malcolm JG, Reinertsen E, Hadjipanayis CG. Spinal cord ependymoma: a review of the literature and case series of ten patients. J Neurooncol 2016;128(3):377–386

33. Chen SC, Kuo PL. Bone metastasis from renal cell carcinoma. Int J Mol Sci 2016;17(6):17
34. Ju DG, Yurter A, Gokaslan ZL, Sciubba DM. Diagnosis and surgical management of breast cancer metastatic to the spine. World J Clin Oncol 2014;5(3):263–271
35. Kushchayeva YS, Kushchayev SV, Wexler JA, et al. Current treatment modalities for spinal metastases secondary to thyroid carcinoma. Thyroid 2014;24(10):1443–1455
36. Vicent S, Perurena N, Govindan R, Lecanda F. Bone metastases in lung cancer. Potential novel approaches to therapy. Am J Respir Crit Care Med 2015;192(7):799–809
37. Amato RJ. Current immunotherapeutic strategies in renal cell carcinoma. Surg Oncol Clin N Am 2007;16(4):975–986, xi–xii
38. Bilsky MH, Laufer I, Fourney DR, et al. Reliability analysis of the epidural spinal cord compression scale. J Neurosurg Spine 2010;13(3):324–328
39. Escudier B, Szczylik C, Porta C, Gore M. Treatment selection in metastatic renal cell carcinoma: expert consensus. Nat Rev Clin Oncol 2012;9(6):327–337
40. Laufer I, Rubin DG, Lis E, et al. The NOMS framework: approach to the treatment of spinal metastatic tumors. Oncologist 2013;18(6):744–751

# 15 Spinal Infections

*Ankur S. Narain, Fady Y. Hijji, Philip K. Louie, Daniel D. Bohl, and Kern Singh*

## 15.1 Introduction

Spinal infections require early diagnosis in order to prevent both structural and neurologic compromises. The differential diagnoses related to symptoms associated with infection include degenerative disease, neoplasm, trauma, and vascular compromise. As such, knowledge of the specific clinical and imaging findings associated with infectious etiologies of the spine is crucial to ensure timely recognition of disease presentation and initiation of treatment (**Table 15.1**).

## 15.2 Vertebral Osteomyelitis and Diskitis

• Background and etiology:
  - Infection of the vertebral body or intervertebral disk.
  - Most commonly caused by hematogenous spread of *Staphylococcus* or *Streptococcus* spp.

**Table 15.1** Summary of infections

| Infection | Presentation | Clinical evaluation | Imaging evaluation | Primary treatment |
|---|---|---|---|---|
| Vertebral osteomyelitis and diskitis | • Axial pain<br>• Fever<br>• Neurologic symptoms | • WBC, ESR, CRP<br>• Blood cultures<br>• UA, urine | • MRI: edema and fluid within disk space | • IV antibiotics 6–8 weeks |
| Spinal epidural abscess | • Axial pain<br>• Motor weakness<br>• Pain | • WBC, ESR, CRP<br>• Blood cultures<br>• Open biopsy | • MRI: fluid within the epidural space | • Surgical with adjuvant antibiotics |
| Spinal TB | • Insidious onset<br>• Paraplegia<br>• Spinal deformity<br>• Back pain | • ESR, CRP<br>• Blood culture<br>• PPD<br>• AFB stain | • MRI: destruction of vertebral bodies with disk sparing<br>• CXR: pulmonary disease | • 6–12 months of multidrug antibiotic therapy |
| Surgical site/postoperative infection | • Erythema<br>• Fluctuance<br>• Drainage from incision | • ESR, CRP, WBC<br>• Wound culture | • CT: abscesses<br>• MRI: fluid collections | • Prophylactic antibiotics<br>• Open irrigation and debridement with antibiotics |

Abbreviations: AFB, acid-fast bacilli; CRP, C-reactive protein; CT, computed tomography; CXR, chest X-ray; ESR, erythrocyte sedimentation rate; IV, intravenous; MRI, magnetic resonance imaging; PPD, purified protein derivatives; TB, tuberculosis; UA, urinalysis; WBC, white blood cell.

- Spread from vascular end plates to:
  - Avascular disk space (diskitis).
  - Vertebral bodies (osteomyelitis).
- Most commonly affects lumbar (58%) > thoracic (30%) > cervical (11%) vertebrae.
- Risk factors include diabetes mellitus, intravenous drug use, corticosteroid therapy.
- Presentation:
  - Common symptoms include axial pain (86%) and fever (35–60%).
  - Neurologic symptoms (34%):
    - Radiculopathy, limb weakness, dysesthesia, urinary retention.
- Clinical evaluation:
  - Inquire about constitutional symptoms, travel history, recent spinal procedures with or without instrumentation.
  - Labs:
    - White blood cell (WBC), erythrocyte sedimentation rate (ESR), C-reactive protein (CRP).
      - ESR and CRP highly specific (98–100%).
      - CRP correlates with response to treatment.
    - Blood cultures:
      - Positive in 58% of cases.
    - Urinalysis and urine culture:
      - To determine if urinary tract infection (UTI) is a source of the primary infection.
- Radiographic evaluation:
  - Plain radiographs: findings occur several weeks after infection onset:
    - Regional osteopenia, periosteal reaction/thickening, focal bone lysis or cortical loss, endosteal scalloping, loss of bony trabeculae.
  - Magnetic resonance imaging (MRI; 94% sensitivity): preferred imaging modality if neurologic deficit is present:
    - T2-weighted imaging shows edema and fluid within disks and adjacent soft tissue (**Fig. 15.1**).
  - Computed tomography (CT) scan (94% sensitivity): performed if MRI contraindicated:
    - Superior to plain radiographs and MRI at analyzing bony margins and identifying involucrum/sequestrum.
  - Bone scan (67% sensitivity): positive within a few days of symptom onset, nonspecific.
- Treatment:
  - Medical treatment:
    - Preferred initial therapeutic option.
    - Intravenous (IV) antibiotics for 6 to 8 weeks, initial broad coverage with narrowing to pathogen-specific regimen pending susceptibilities.
  - Surgical therapy:
    - Indications:
      - Failure of medical management.
      - Drainage of abscesses and debridement of infected tissue.
      - Development of neurological deterioration.
      - Decompression of neural structures.
      - Spinal instability.

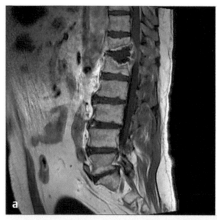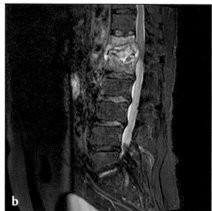

**Fig. 15.1 (a)** Sagittal T1-weighted MRI showing osteomyelitis involving the T12–L1 disk space, vertebral bodies, and surrounding soft tissue. **(b)** Sagittal T2-weighted MRI showing osteomyelitis involving the T12–L1 disk space, vertebral bodies, and surrounding soft tissue.

## 15.3 Spinal Epidural Abscess

- Background and etiology:
  - Infection of the epidural space.
  - Source:
    - Direct inoculation.
    - Contiguous spread:
      - Adjacent osteomyelitis or diskitis.
    - Hematogenous extension.
  - *S. aureus* is the most common pathogen (64%).
  - Affects lumbar (48%) > thoracic (31–33%) > cervical (22–24%) spine.
  - Risk factors: intravenous drug use (IVDU; 22–23%), diabetes mellitus (27–28%).
- Presentation:
  - Most common symptoms include axial pain (67%), neuromuscular complaints (52%), fever (44%).
  - Large lesions can compress neural elements and lead to focal neurologic deficits.
- Clinical evaluation:
  - Labs:
    - WBC, ESR, CRP.
    - Blood cultures.
  - Possible open biopsy to identify specific organism.
- Radiographic evaluation:
  - Plain radiographs: may show disk narrowing and/or bone lysis.
  - MRI (high sensitivity and specificity): clearly demonstrates fluid collection within the epidural space (**Fig. 15.2**).
- Treatment:
  - Surgical intervention with adjuvant antibiotics:
    - Indicated if neurologic deficit is present.

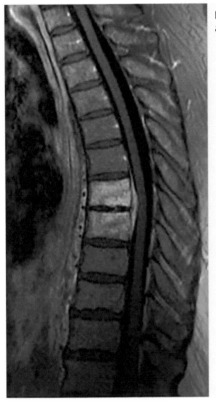

**Fig. 15.2** Sagittal T1-weighted MRI showing an epidural abscess in the thoracic spine.

- Irrigation and debridement with neurologic decompression.
- Approach based on location and etiology:
  - Posterior: laminectomy.
  - Anterior: ventral abscess or vertebral osteomyelitis.
- Arthrodesis if instability suspected.
  - Medical therapy with antibiotics only:
    - Indicated if neurologic deficits are absent.
    - High conversion rate to surgical therapy (10–49%).

# 15.4  Spinal Tuberculosis (Pott's Disease)

- Background and etiology:
  - Granulomatous infection of the spine.
  - Distant source or latent reactivation leads to inoculation within the peridiskal metaphysis of the vertebral end plate:
    - Inflammatory response leads to caseating granuloma formation.
    - Active bone destruction (spondylosis).
    - Often spreads via the anterior longitudinal ligament to nearby levels.

- Spine is the most common site of skeletal tuberculosis (TB) involvement (1% of all TB cases, 50% of those with musculoskeletal involvement):
  ◦ Thoracic and upper lumbar levels most commonly affected.
- Presentation:
  - Insidious progression of disease over weeks to years.
  - Paraplegia and spinal deformity (70%):
    ◦ Kyphosis due to anterior vertebral body collapse.
  - Back pain.
  - Constitutional complaints.
  - Symptoms of pulmonary TB:
    ◦ Persistent cough, hemoptysis.
- Clinical evaluation:
  - Inquire about current TB infection or previous TB exposure.
  - Labs:
    ◦ ESR, CRP, blood cultures.
    ◦ Tuberculin purified protein derivative (PPD) skin test.
    ◦ Sputum, bone tissue, abscess aspirate for acid-fast bacilli stain:
      ▪ Abscess aspirates obtained via CT- or ultrasound-guided biopsy.
- Radiographic evaluation:
  - Chest X-ray: to evaluate for pulmonary disease, extensive bony lesions, focal kyphosis.
  - Plain radiography: findings require more than 30% of vertebral body destruction; can be delayed up to 6 months after infection:
    ◦ Reduction in vertebral height often with irregularity of the anterosuperior end plate.
    ◦ Subligamentous extension with further progression, resulting in irregularity at the anterior vertebral margin.
  - MRI (highly sensitive and specific): destruction of vertebral bodies with intervertebral disk sparing:
    ◦ T1: hypointense marrow in adjacent vertebrae (**Fig. 15.3a**).
    ◦ T2: hyperintense marrow, disk, soft-tissue involvement (**Fig. 15.3b**).
- Treatment:
  - Medical therapy:
    ◦ Multidrug treatment of 6 to 12 months:
      ▪ Rifampin.
      ▪ Pyrazinamide.
      ▪ Streptomycin or ethambutol.
      ▪ Isoniazid.
  - Surgical therapy:
    ◦ Indications:
      ▪ Failure of medical therapy.
      ▪ Instability.
      ▪ Deformity.
      ▪ Neurologic decline.
      ▪ Intractable pain caused by abscess.
    ◦ Anterior reconstruction ± supplemental posterior fixation to prevent deformity.

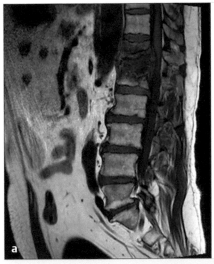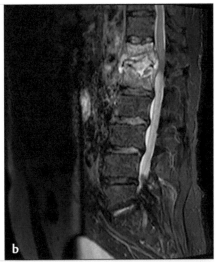

**Fig. 15.3 (a)** Sagittal T1-weighted MRI showing spinal TB infection involving T12–L1. **(b)** Sagittal T2-weighted MRI showing spinal TB infection involving T12–L1.

# 15.5 Surgical Site and Postoperative Infections

- Background and etiology:
  - Direct inoculation of exposed wound by skin flora.
  - Occurs in 0.7 to 12% of spinal operations in adults:
    ◦ Leads to increased morbidity, mortality, health care costs.
  - Risk factors include diabetes, previous surgical site infection, spinal deformity, longer operative times, multiple-level fusion, posterior surgical approaches, combined anteroposterior surgical approaches, estimated blood loss greater than 1 L.
- Presentation:
  - Location:
    ◦ Superficial: contained within the skin and subcutaneous tissues without fascial involvement (suprafascial).
    ◦ Deep: deep to the lumbodorsal fascia (lumbar) or ligamentum nuchae (cervical).
  - Erythema, palpable fluctuance, drainage from the incision.
- Clinical evaluation:
  - Labs:
    ◦ ESR, CRP, WBC.
  - Wound culture:
    ◦ Intraoperative cultures are best.
    ◦ Deep cultures are best since they are not contaminated with skin flora.

- Radiographic evaluation:
  - Plain radiographs: often without obvious abnormalities.
  - CT scan: reveals abscesses.
  - MRI: superior soft-tissue resolution allows for enhanced views of fluid collections (**Figs. 15.4, 15.5**).
- Treatment:
  - Prevention:
    ○ Prophylactic antibiotics within 60 minutes prior to procedure start.
    ○ Redosing if the procedure is prolonged (~3–4 hours).
  - Irrigation and debridement with subsequent 6-week course of antibiotics:
    ○ Collect intraoperative deep wound cultures before antibiotic administration.

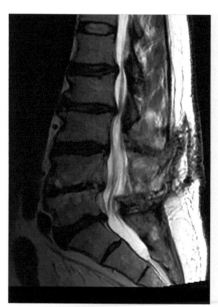

**Fig. 15.4** Sagittal STIR-weighted MRI showing postoperative infection at the lumbosacral junction with soft-tissue involvement.

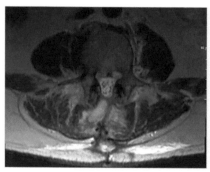

**Fig. 15.5** Axial T2-weighted MRI showing postoperative infection extending into posterior musculature.

# Suggested Readings

1. Ansari S, Amanullah MF, Ahmad K, Rauniyar RK. Pott's spine: diagnostic imaging modalities and technology advancements. N Am J Med Sci 2013;5(7):404–411
2. Arko L IV, Quach E, Nguyen V, Chang D, Sukul V, Kim BS. Medical and surgical management of spinal epidural abscess: a systematic review. Neurosurg Focus 2014;37(2):E4
3. Kilborn T, Janse van Rensburg P, Candy S. Pediatric and adult spinal tuberculosis: imaging and pathophysiology. Neuroimaging Clin N Am 2015;25(2):209–231
4. Mazzie JP, Brooks MK, Gnerre J. Imaging and management of postoperative spine infection. Neuroimaging Clin N Am 2014;24(2):365–374
5. Mylona E, Samarkos M, Kakalou E, Fanourgiakis P, Skoutelis A. Pyogenic vertebral osteomyelitis: a systematic review of clinical characteristics. Semin Arthritis Rheum 2009;39(1):10–17
6. Pull ter Gunne AF, Cohen DB. Incidence, prevalence, and analysis of risk factors for surgical site infection following adult spinal surgery. Spine 2009;34(13):1422–1428
7. Suppiah S, Meng Y, Fehlings MG, Massicotte EM, Yee A, Shamji MF. How best to manage the spinal epidural abscess? A current systematic review. World Neurosurg 2016;93:20–28
8. Zimmerli W. Clinical practice. Vertebral osteomyelitis. N Engl J Med 2010;362(11):1022–1029

# 16 Pediatrics

*Jonathan Markowitz, Ankur S. Narain, Fady Y. Hijji, Philip K. Louie, Daniel D. Bohl, and Kern Singh*

## 16.1 Background

- Most congenital spinal pathologies affect the upper cervical or lumbar regions:
  - Due to defective spina cord embryogenesis and/or vertebral malformation.
- Neural tube defect (NTD):
  - Incomplete fusion of the neural tube during fetal development.
  - Myelodysplasia is the most common type of NTD:
    - These include spina bifida occulta, meningocele, myelomeningocele, and rachischisis.
- Spine bifida affects approximately 1,500 births annually in the United States:
  - Highest rates of NTDs are found in China, Ireland, Great Britain, Pakistan, India, and Egypt.

## 16.2 Myelodysplasia (Spina Bifida)

- Background and etiology:
  - Incomplete closure of the caudal end of the neural tube during spinal cord development and lack of fusion of vertebral arches:
    - Development of the vertebrae and spinal column begin in the third week of embryonic development.
    - The neural tube is created by the inward folding and fusing of the neural plate (primary neurulation).
    - Neural tube is the embryo's precursor to the central nervous system.
  - Results in an open lesion or sac (spina bifida cystica) that can contain the spinal cord, nerve roots, and meninges:
    - Varying degrees of myelodysplasia depending on level of failed closure.
  - Environmental causes:
    - Maternal folic acid deficiency.
    - Maternal use of folic acid antagonists (dihydrofolate reductase inhibitors): aminopterin, methotrexate, sulfasalazine, pyrimethamine, triamterene, and trimethoprim.
    - Antiepileptic drugs: carbamazepine, valproate, phenytoin, primidone, and phenobarbital.
    - Maternal hyperthermia.
    - Maternal diabetes.

- Types of myelodysplasia:
  - Spina bifida occulta:
    - Mildest form.
    - Unfused vertebral arch.
    - Meninges do not herniate through the opening in the spinal canal.
  - Meningocele:
    - A subset of spina bifida cystica:
      - Spinal elements are contained within a sac.
    - Herniation of the meninges (excluding the spinal cord), through the opening in the spinal canal.
  - Myelomeningocele:
    - A subset of spina bifida cystica.
    - Herniation of the meninges and the spinal cord through the opening in the spinal canal.
  - Rachischisis:
    - Neural elements exposed with no covering.
- Presentation:
  - Mild forms (i.e., spina bifida occulta) may be asymptomatic:
    - Occasional abnormal tuft of hair or small dimple at the site of the spinal malformation.
  - Meningocele or myelomeningocele will present with a cyst containing neural elements.
  - Neurological symptoms can include bladder, motor, and sensory paralysis below the level of the spinal lesion.
  - Often associated with latex allergy.
  - Functional status is primarily related to the level of the defect (**Table 16.1**):

**Table 16.1** Clinical presentation associated with level of myelodysplasia

| Level | Hip deformity | Knee deformity | Foot deformity | Degree of ambulation[a] | Muscles involved | Orthosis |
|---|---|---|---|---|---|---|
| L1 | Flexion/ external rotation | – | Equinovarus | Nonambulatory | – | HKAFO |
| L2 | Flexion/ adduction | Flexion | Equinovarus | Nonambulatory | Quadriceps | HKAFO |
| L3 | Flexion/ adduction | Recurva- tum | Equinovarus | Household | Iliopsoas and hip adductors | KAFO |
| L4 | Flexion/ adduction | Extension | Cavovarus | Household, some community | Quadriceps and tibialis anterior | AFO |
| L5 | Flexed | Limited flexion | Calcaneal valgus | Community | EHL, EDL and gluteus medius and minimus | AFO |
| S1 | – | – | Foot deformity | Normal | Gastrocsoleus | Shoes |

Abbreviations: AFO, ankle–foot orthosis; EDL, extensor digitorum longus; EHL, extensor hallucis longus; HKAFO, hip–knee–ankle–foot orthosis; KAFO, knee–ankle–foot orthosis.
Note: Level of myelodysplastic defect and corresponding deformity and functional status.
[a]Community ambulation defined as locomotion outdoors that includes activities necessary to live independently.

- ○ Deformities that occur in patients with myelomeningocele are secondary to unbalanced/asymmetric muscle action around joints, paralysis, and decreased sensation in the lower extremities.
- ○ Lesion of L3 or above are mostly confined to a wheelchair.
  - – Changes in functional level should alert the physician to the possibility of tethered cord syndrome:
    - ○ Formation of fibrous attachments between the spinal cord and spinal canal:
      - ▪ Results in stretching of the spinal cord and progressive cord damage and neurologic deficit.
- Clinical evaluation:
  - – Examination should include assessment of level and degree of motor and sensory function, range of motion (ROM), spinal deformity, integrity of the skin, and associated deformities and contractures.
  - – Prenatal laboratory diagnosis:
    - ○ Maternal screening of serum alpha fetoprotein (AFP) levels:
      - ▪ Performed ideally at 16 to 18 weeks of gestation, but can be performed as early as 15 weeks or as late as 20 weeks.
      - ▪ First trimester screening is not recommended because of low sensitivity.
  - – Magnetic resonance imaging (MRI) or computed tomography (CT) may be performed to get a more precise understanding of the underlying defect (**Fig. 16.1**):
    - ○ Dysplasia of the spinal cord and nerve roots may lead to bowel, bladder, motor, and sensory paralysis below the level of the lesion.
- Treatment and prevention:
  - – Maternal consumption of 0.4 mg (400 µg) of folic acid a day for ≥3 months before conception, decrease the chance of NTD by 70 to 80%.
  - – Aim of treatment is to enable the child to reach the highest degree of strength, function, and independence:
    - ○ Spina bifida occulta:
      - ▪ Patients usually do not need surgery.
      - ▪ Conservative management and watchful monitoring is recommended.
    - ○ Meningocele:
      - ▪ Surgical treatment for the removal of the cyst is typically recommended.
      - ▪ If later orthopedic surgical intervention is necessary, it usually focuses on balancing of the muscles and correction of deformities.
    - ○ Myelomeningocele and rachischisis:
      - ▪ Early treatment with antibiotics is necessary in order to prevent infection of the spinal cord.
      - ▪ Requires surgery within the first few days of life to correct the spinal defect and prevent infection and further injury to the exposed spinal cord/nerve roots.
      - ▪ Most common complications with surgery are tethered spinal cord and hydrocephalus.
      - ▪ In utero surgical intervention may be considered.

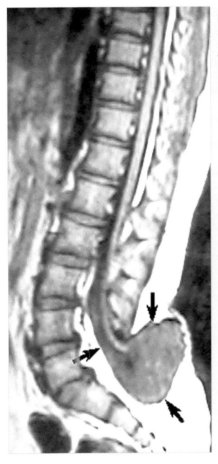

**Fig. 16.1** Sagittal T1-weighted MRI demonstrating myelomeningocele contiguous with spinal canal contents (*arrows*). (Reproduced with permission from Khanna AJ, ed. MRI Essentials for the Spine Specialist. New York, NY: Thieme; 2014.)

# 16.3 Congenital Torticollis

- Background and etiology:
  - Contracture of the sternocleidomastoid (SCM).
  - 0.3 to 2% of newborns.
  - More common in males (1.5:1).
  - Etiology unknown:
    - Possibly due to malposition of the head in utero and injury to the SCM muscle resulting in fibrosis.
  - Usually evident by 2 to 4 weeks of age:
    - Not to be confused with acquired, which usually occurs due to injury, inflammation, or medications.
  - Three types of congenital torticollis:
    - Postural: no muscle tightness or restriction to passive ROM, but infant has a postural preference.

- ◦ Muscular: tightness of SCM with limitation in passive ROM.
- ◦ SCM mass: palpable pseudotumor or swelling in the body of SCM, limited in passive ROM.
- Clinical presentation:
  - Characterized by lateral neck flexion (head tilted to affected side) and neck rotation (chin pointed to contralateral side):
    - ◦ Reduced cervical ROM.
    - ◦ Infant usually has a preferred head position during feeding and sleeping.
    - ◦ Right SCM more commonly affected.
  - Associated with facial asymmetry.
- Clinical evaluation and imaging:
  - A diagnosis of congenital muscular torticollis can be made on the basis of history and physical examination.
- Treatment:
  - Nonoperative treatment:
    - ◦ Passive stretching exercises:
      - ▪ Rotate infant's chin to ipsilateral shoulder while simultaneously tilting the head toward so that the ear touches the contralateral shoulder.
    - ◦ Adjunctive use of soft cervical collar.
  - Surgical treatment:
    - ◦ Recommended when patient has persistently restricted ROM.
    - ◦ Lengthens the contracted SCM through a unipolar release, bipolar release, endoscopic release, and subperiosteal lengthening.
    - ◦ Postoperative physical therapy consisting of ROM exercises.
    - ◦ A cervical collar may be worn postoperatively.

# 16.4 Klippel–Feil Syndrome

- Background and etiology:
  - Congenital skeletal disorder characterized by abnormal union or fusion of two or more cervical vertebrae:
    - ◦ Failure of normal segmentation or formation of cervical vertebrae precursors at 3 to 8 weeks.
- Classification:
  - No universally agreed upon classification system.
  - Samartzis' classification system:
    - ◦ Type I: single-level fusion.
    - ◦ Type II: multiple, noncontiguous fused segments.
    - ◦ Type III: multiple, contiguous fused segments.
- Clinical presentation:
  - Classic triad (seen in <50% of cases):
    - ◦ Short neck.

- ○ Low posterior hairline.
- ○ Decreased cervical ROM.
  - Commonly associated with other congenital abnormalities (**Table 16.2**).
  - Degenerative cervical disk disease is seen in almost 100% of patients.
- Clinical evaluation and imaging:
  - Radiographs and CT: anteroposterior (AP)/axial, lateral/sagittal, and odontoid views of cervical spine (**Fig. 16.2**):
    - ○ Fusion of at least two cervical vertebrae.
  - Consider MRI to rule out intraspinal cord abnormalities.
- Treatment and prevention:
  - Conservative management.
  - Avoid contact sports.
  - If patient has chronic pain and/or myelopathy, surgical decompression and fusion is recommended.

**Table 16.2** Spectrum of anomalies known to be associated with Klippel-Feil syndrome

| Anomaly | Percentage of patients |
| --- | --- |
| Congenital scoliosis | >50 |
| Sensorineural hearing impairment | 30 |
| Genitourinary abnormalities | 25–35 |
| Sprengel's deformity | 20–30 |
| Facial asymmetry | 20 |
| Torticollis | 20 |
| Ptosis, horizontal nystagmus, and cleft palate | Common |

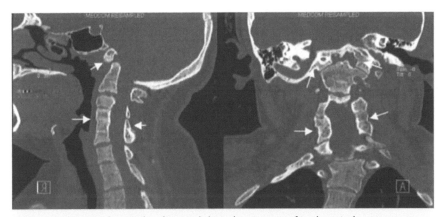

**Fig. 16.2** CT scan of sagittal and coronal slices demonstrates fused cervical segments (*arrows*), indicating Klippel–Feil syndrome.

## Suggested Readings

1.  Frey L, Hauser WA. Epidemiology of neural tube defects. Epilepsia 2003;44 (Suppl 3):4–13
2.  Centers for Disease Control (CDC). Economic burden of spina bifida: United States, 1980-1990. Morb Mortal Wkly Rep 1989;38(15):264–267
3.  Shaer CM, Chescheir N, Schulkin J. Myelomeningocele: a review of the epidemiology, genetics, risk factors for conception, prenatal diagnosis, and prognosis for affected individuals. Obstet Gynecol Surv 2007;62(7):471–479
4.  Nilesh K, Mukherji S. Congenital muscular torticollis. Ann Maxillofac Surg 2013;3(2):198–200
5.  Tomczak KK, Rosman NP. Torticollis. J Child Neurol 2013;28(3):365–378
6.  Das BK, Matin A, Roy RR, Islam MR, Islam R, Khan R. Congenital muscular torticollis: A descriptive study of 16 cases. Bangladesh J Child Health. 2010;34(3):92–98
7.  Tracy MR, Dormans JP, Kusumi K. Klippel-Feil syndrome: clinical features and current understanding of etiology. Clin Orthop Relat Res 2004;(424):183–190

# 17 Anterior Cervical Diskectomy and Fusion

*Ankur S. Narain, Fady Y. Hijji, Philip K. Louie, Daniel D. Bohl, and Kern Singh*

## 17.1 Case Presentation: Presentation and Preoperative Imaging

A 38-year-old man presents to the office with long-standing neck pain radiating into the bilateral upper extremities. He notes numbness and tingling in the forearms bilaterally. He also has weakness along with decreased grip strength and upper extremity dexterity bilaterally. He denies any recent trauma or infections. Conservative therapy with home exercises, nonsteroidal anti-inflammatory drugs (NSAIDs), and oral steroids have only provided temporary relief.

## 17.2 Indications

• Symptomatic cervical disk herniation with radiculopathy or myelopathy (**Fig. 17.1**).
• Cervical spondylosis with radiculopathy or myelopathy.
• Ossification of the posterior longitudinal ligament present with myelopathy.
• Unstable cervical fractures.

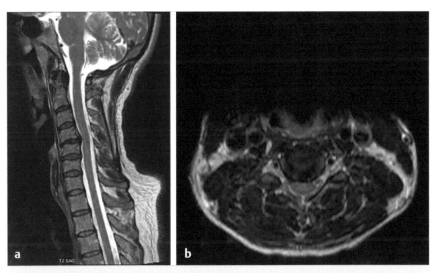

**Fig. 17.1 (a,b)** Sagittal and axial T2-weighted MRI demonstrating a herniated nucleus pulposus at C4–C5 with spinal cord compression.

## 17.3 Positioning

- Supine.
- Superficial landmarks include the following:
  - Lower border of mandible (C2–C3.)
  - Hyoid bone (C3).
  - Thyroid cartilage (C4–C5).
  - Cricoid cartilage (C6).

## 17.4 Approach

- Superficial dissection:
  - Skin incision at the level of pathology: oblique from midline to the posterior border of the sternocleidomastoid (SCM):
    ◦ Incise the fascial sheath over the platysma; split the platysma longitudinally
    ◦ No internervous plane is present as the platysma, which is innervated by the facial nerve, is divided beneath the fascial sheath.
  - Identify the anterior border of the SCM and incise the fascia immediately anterior to it; gently retract the SCM laterally .
  - Retract the strap muscles and tracheoesophageal structures medially. An internervous plane is present between the SCM (CN XI) and the strap muscles (C1–C3).
- Deep dissection:
  - The carotid sheath is now exposed; develop a plane between the carotid sheath and midline structures.
  - Retract the carotid sheath and SCM laterally.
  - After development of a plane deep to the pretracheal fascia, the cervical vertebrae should be visible.
  - Split the longus colli muscles longitudinally (**Fig. 17.2**):
    ◦ The recurrent laryngeal nerve is at risk during this approach; protect it with placement of retractors under the medial edge of the longus colli.

## 17.5 Implants and Hardware

- Structural bone grafts are placed after the diskectomy is performed:
  - Bone grafts can be auto- or allograft.
  - Grafts can also be alternative materials such as polyetheretherketone (PEEK) or carbon fiber filled with local bone obtained from the osteophyte resection or from bone graft substitutes.
- Anterior cervical plate and screws are used to stabilize the vertebral levels directly adjacent to the resected disk space.

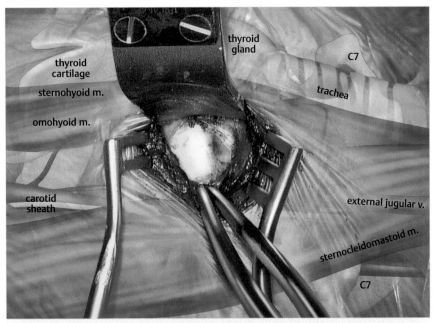

**Fig. 17.2** Top-down view. Deep exposure showing the exposed vertebral body and adjacent disk spaces after retraction of the longus colli muscles. (Reproduced with permission from Singh K, Vaccaro AR, eds. Pocket Atlas of Spine Surgery. 2nd ed. New York, NY: Thieme; 2018.)

# 17.6 Case Presentation: Postoperative Imaging and Outcome

The patient underwent a C4–C5 anterior cervical diskectomy and fusion (ACDF) with placement of an interbody graft, anterior plate, and screw instrumentation. At 6-month follow-up, the patient reported minimal neck pain, with greatly reduced numbness and tingling in the bilateral upper extremities. Postoperative computed tomography (CT) and plain radiographs demonstrated adequately placed instrumentation with solid bony fusion at 6 months postoperatively (**Fig. 17.3**).

## 17.6.1 Complications

- Horner's syndrome:
  - Due to irritation of the sympathetic nerves or stellate ganglion:
    - Most commonly associated with cervical retractors that are placed above the longus coli.
  - Presents with ptosis, anhydrosis, miosis, and loss of ciliospinal reflex.
- Hoarseness:
  - Irritation to the recurrent laryngeal nerve.

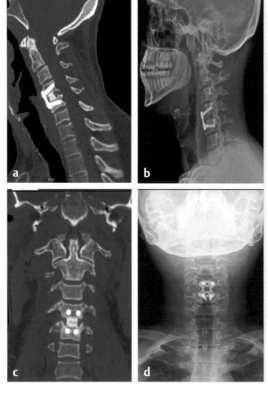

**Fig. 17.3 (a,b)** Sagittal postoperative CT and plain radiograph images demonstrating placement of anterior cage and screw instrumentation with bony fusion. **(c,d)** Coronal and anteroposterior postoperative CT and plain radiograph images demonstrating proper screw placement with bony fusion.

- Prevention:
  ◦ Place retractors under the medial edge of the longus colli.
• Dysphagia:
  - Caused by excessive retraction of the esophagus:
    ◦ Most commonly associated with increased operative time, number of surgical levels, and exposures at C3–C4 and C7–T1.
    ◦ Not associated with side of surgical exposure (i.e., right vs. left).
  - Prevention:
    ◦ Intermittent relaxation of self-retaining retractors during the procedure, partially deflating the endotracheal cuff once the cervical retractors are in position.
• Retropharyngeal hematoma:
  - Presents with respiratory difficulty and a tense neck mass.
  - Prevention:
    ◦ Placement of a cervical drain in those at risk (older age, smoking history, increased operative levels).
  - Treatment:
    ◦ Requires emergent decompression.

# 18 Posterior Cervical Laminoplasty with Instrumentation

*Ankur S. Narain, Fady Y. Hijji, Philip K. Louie, Daniel D. Bohl, and Kern Singh*

## 18.1 Case Presentation

A 70-year-old man presents to the clinic complaining of worsening ambulation. He also notes the pain radiates to his left scapula and left arm and is associated with numbness and paresthesia of his left lateral forearm and thumb. He also notes weakness and difficulty with fine motor tasks such as buttoning his shirt. On physical examination, the patient exhibits decreased sensation of his left lateral forearm, thumb, and index finger. He exhibits full strength on shoulder abduction, elbow flexion and extension, and wrist flexion and extension. He has a positive Spurling test, with a positive Hoffman sign. He is unable to perform the grip release test with 20 cycles of grips and releases within 10 seconds. The patient's radiographs and magnetic resonance imaging (MRI) are provided in **Figs. 18.1** and **18.2**. The patient is subsequently scheduled to receive a posterior cervical laminoplasty with instrumentation from C3 to C6.

## 18.2 Indications

- Paracentral cervical disk herniations.
- Cervical spinal stenosis at multiple levels.
- Cervical tumors.

## 18.3 Positioning

- Prone.
- Landmarks:
  - Spinous processes:

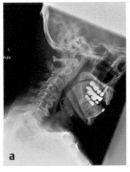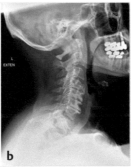

**Fig. 18.1** Flexion **(a)** and extension **(b)** of cervical radiographs. There is significant cervical spondylosis of C3–T1 with C3–C4 and C7–T1 spondylolisthesis.

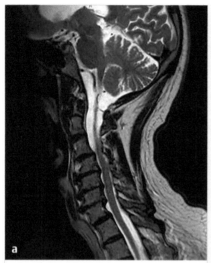

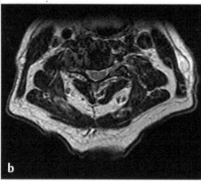

**Fig. 18.2** Sagittal **(a)** and axial T2-weighted **(b)** cervical MRI. There is C3–T1 spondylosis with moderate to severe spinal stenosis.

- ○ C2, C7, and T1 are largest spinous processes in the cervical region.
- ○ C7 and T1 difficult to differentiate via palpation.

# 18.4  Approach

## 18.4.1  Superficial Dissection

- The skin incision is made midline over the targeted cervical levels:
  - Intraoperative imaging and needle placement is necessary to confirm the correct level of decompression.
  - The internervous plane is located between the paraspinal cervical muscles of either side. The dorsal rami of the cervical roots supply this region.
- The paracervical muscles are stripped subperiosteally to avoid bleeding:
  - Only the medial portion of the lamina/facet junction is exposed.

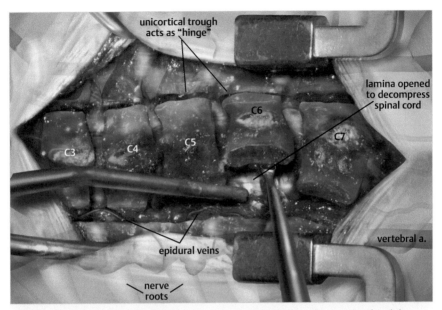

**Fig. 18.3** Top-down view. A bicortical and unicortical trough have been created and the lamina has been opened to decompress the spinal cord. (Reproduced with permission from Singh K, Vaccaro AR, eds. Pocket Atlas of Spine Surgery. 2nd ed. New York, NY: Thieme; 2018.)

## 18.4.2  Deep Dissection

- Spinous processes are removed for the desired levels.
- The junction between the lamina and facets is identified and an opening is created (**Fig. 18.3**):
  - This opening is bicortical and penetrates completely through the bone.
- A similar trough is made on the contralateral side; however, this side is unicortical:
  - Serves as a hinge.

## 18.5  Implants and Hardware

- The lamina is lifted using the unicortical trough as a hinge.
- Plates are secured to the free end into the lateral mass (**Fig. 18.4**).

## 18.6  Case Presentation: Postoperative Outcome, and Imaging

The patient underwent a C3 to C6 posterior cervical laminoplasty with instrumentation. At 6-week follow-up, the patient notes significant improvement in his pain and complete resolution of his sensory and motor deficits. Postoperative radiographs demonstrate appropriate instrument positioning (**Fig. 18.5**).

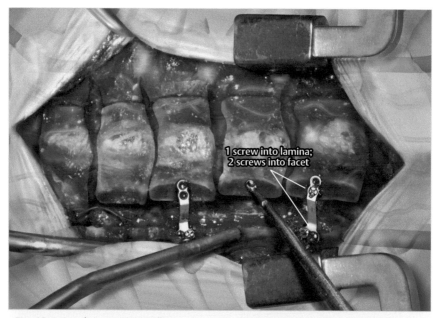

**Fig. 18.4** Top-down view. A midline exposure has been performed with subperiosteal elevation of the paracervical muscles up the medial facet joints. (Reproduced with permission from Singh K, Vaccaro AR, eds. Pocket Atlas of Spine Surgery. 2nd ed. New York, NY: Thieme; 2018.)

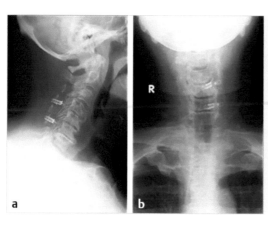

**Fig. 18.5** Lateral **(a)** and anteroposterior **(b)** radiographs. Six-week postoperative radiographs following posterior cervical laminoplasty demonstrating instrumentation placed at the C4 and C6 laminae.

# 18.7 Complications

- C5 nerve root palsy:
  - Incidence of 0.5 to 13.3%.
  - Unclear etiology:
    - Thought to be due to posterior translation of the spinal cord following decompression:

- ▪ The short C5 nerve root experiences subsequent stretching.
  - ○ No clear method for avoidance at this time.
- Risk factors:
  - ○ Associated with significant spinal cord rotation.
  - ○ Excessive posterior spinal cord drift.
  - ○ Narrow foramina.
  - ○ Ossified posterior longitudinal ligament.
- Presents with:
  - ○ Biceps and deltoid weakness.
  - ○ Sensory loss of the lateral upper arm.
  - ○ Presents 48 to 72 hours following surgery.
- Treatment:
  - ○ Self-limited; most resolve within 6 months.
• Postoperative neck pain and stiffness:
  - Incidence of 40 to 60% and 20 to 50% for neck pain and stiffness, respectively. However, this incidence is based upon older literature where patients were immobilized for 6 to 12 weeks postoperatively.
  - Unclear etiology:
    - ○ Attributed to excessive paracervical periosteal stripping and postoperative immobilization.
  - Risk factors:
    - ○ Intraoperative facet joint disruption.
  - Prevention:
    - ○ Maintaining exposure medial to the facet capsules to avoid direct damage.
• Postoperative hematoma:
  - Damage to thin-walled epidural vessels in the cervical canal can result in excessive bleeding.
  - Treatment:
    - ○ Control bleeding with hemostatic sponges intraoperatively.
  - Prevention:
    - ○ Obtain adequate hemostasis prior to closure.
    - ○ Placement of wound drains while routinely performed may not prevent the formation of a hematoma.

## Suggested Readings

1. Ratliff JK, Cooper PR. Cervical laminoplasty: a critical review. J Neurosurg 2003;98(3, Suppl):230–238
2. Gu Y, Cao P, Gao R, et al. Incidence and risk factors of C5 palsy following posterior cervical decompression: a systematic review. PLoS One 2014;9(8):e101933
3. Hosono N, Yonenobu K, Ono K. Neck and shoulder pain after laminoplasty. A noticeable complication. Spine 1996;21(17):1969–1973

# 19 Posterior Cervical Laminectomy and Fusion

*Ankur S. Narain, Fady Y. Hijji, Philip K. Louie, Daniel D. Bohl, and Kern Singh*

## 19.1 Case Presentation and Preoperative Imaging

A 61-year-old woman presents to your office with chronic neck pain and numbness in her right hand. The numbness is exacerbated by turning her head to the right, looking up, and overhead reaching. She has 5/5 strength and intact reflexes in the upper extremities bilaterally, with no clonus or spasticity. Hoffman's sign is positive bilaterally. Conservative therapy with heat and ice packs, and physical therapy have provided minimal pain relief. Magnetic resonance imaging (MRI) scan of the cervical spine was recommended (**Fig. 19.1**).

## 19.2 Indications

- Degenerative cervical disk disease with central stenosis, neuroforaminal stenosis, or myelopathy.
- Tumor.
- Epidural abscess.
- Ossification of the posterior longitudinal ligament with stenosis.

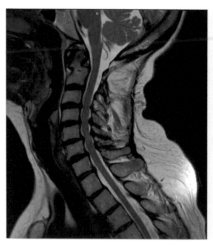

**Fig. 19.1** Sagittal T2-weighted magnetic resonance imaging (MRI) demonstrating central spinal stenosis at C4–C5 and C5–C6.

# 19.3 Positioning

- Prone.
- Landmarks:
  - Spinous processes:
    - C2, C7–T1 are the most prominent.

# 19.4 Approach

- Superficial dissection:
  - Straight incision is made in the midline:
    - Internervous plane is in the midline; paracervical muscles are segmentally innervated by the left and right posterior rami.
    - Minimal bleeding may emanate from the venous plexuses.
  - Dissection is performed through the ligamentum nuchae:
    - Continuous with the supraspinous ligament.
- Deep dissection:
  - Remove paracervical muscles subperiosteally (**Fig. 19.2**):
    - Excessive bleeding may occur from the segmental arterial vessels.
  - Perform laminectomy at the junction between the lamina and lateral mass of each side:
    - The epidural veins are thin and may bleed copiously.

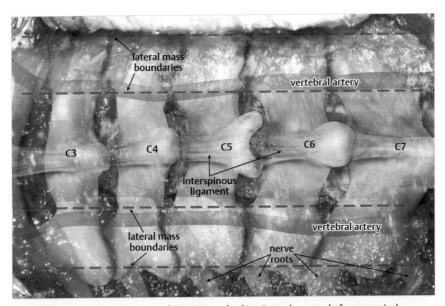

**Fig. 19.2** Top-down view. Deep dissection and subperiosteal removal of paracervical muscles with adequate exposure of the lateral mass's superior, inferior, medial, and lateral borders. (Reproduced with permission from Singh K, Vaccaro AR, eds. Pocket Atlas of Spine Surgery. 2nd ed. New York, NY: Thieme; 2018.)

## 19.5  Implants and Hardware

• Lateral mass screws are placed and connected via rods and cross-connectors.

## 19.6  Case Presentation: Postoperative Imaging and Outcomes

The patient underwent a posterior cervical laminectomy and fusion (PCLF) at C3–C7 with bilateral lateral mass screw instrumentation for fixation. The patient noted significant symptom improvement at 6 months postoperatively, with decreases in pain, numbness, and tingling from her initial presentation. Postoperative radiographs demonstrated adequate placement of instrumentation without evidence of loosening (**Fig. 19.3**).

## 19.7  Complications

• Nerve root injury:
  - Direct damage during foraminotomy or lateral mass screw placement.
  - C5 palsy is the most common (0.5–8%).
  - Prevention:
    ◦ Maintain a cranial and lateral trajectory for screw placement.
  - Treatment:
    ◦ Nerve palsy is usually self-limited and resolves within 6 to 12 months.
• Durotomy:
  - Tear of the dura resultant from direct damage during laminectomy.
  - Presents with orthostatic headache, nausea, vomiting.
  - Prevention:
    ◦ Care should be taken when placing large instruments near the central canal.
  - Treatment:
    ◦ Primary repair with nonabsorbable sutures.
    ◦ Head elevated to reduce pressure on the repair.

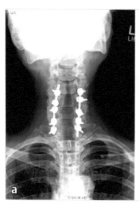 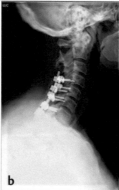

**Fig. 19.3** Anteroposterior **(a)** and lateral **(b)** cervical postoperative radiographs showing posterior cervical laminectomy and fusion with lateral mass screw placement with rod connectors.

- Vertebral artery injury:
  - Often occurs from misdirected lateral mass screws.
  - Presents with hemorrhage, possible central nervous system ischemia.
  - 4-8% incidence.
  - Prevention:
    - Ensure adequate surgical planning via use of preoperative imaging to determine arterial course.
  - Treatment:
    - Aggressive intravenous (IV) fluid resuscitation, placement of the head in a neutral position.
    - Hemostasis via digital pressure, Gelfoam.
    - Definitive surgical interventions: primary repair versus bypass versus sacrifice:
      - Nondominant vertebral artery can often be safely sacrificed without complication.
- Postoperative epidural hematoma:
  - Accumulation of postoperative edema and bleeding.
  - Presents with gradual postoperative neurologic deficit.
  - Risk factors include increasing number of surgical levels, history of coagulopathies or vascular anomalies.
  - Prevention:
    - Placement of subfascial cervical drains prior to closure.

## Suggested Readings

1. Awad JN, Kebaish KM, Donigan J, Cohen DB, Kostuik JP. Analysis of the risk factors for the development of post-operative spinal epidural haematoma. J Bone Joint Surg Br 2005;87(9):1248–1252
2. Schroeder GD, Hsu WK. Vertebral artery injuries in cervical spine surgery. Surg Neurol Int 2013;4(Suppl 5):S362–S367

# 20 Open Posterolateral Lumbar Fusion

*Ankur S. Narain, Fady Y. Hijji, Philip K. Louie, Daniel D. Bohl, and Kern Singh*

## 20.1 Case Presentation

A 59-year-old woman presents to the clinic complaining of a 9-month history of bilateral lower extremity pain and dysesthesias radiating into her right lateral thigh and medial calf. She describes her pain as constant and only improved when leaning forward. She states her pain is worsened with activity including standing and walking for extended periods of time. She denies any improvement in her pain after 6 months of physical therapy and epidural injections. On physical examination, the patient demonstrates weakness in great toe extension in the right foot and sensory deficits at the dorsum of the foot. There is no hyper- or hyporeflexia when eliciting the right Achilles' tendon reflex. The patient's radiographs and magnetic resonance imaging (MRI) are presented in **Figs. 20.1, 20.2.** The patient was scheduled to undergo an open posterolateral lumbar fusion (PLF) of the L4–L5 interspace.

## 20.2 Indications

- Lumbar nerve root compression.
- Lumbar instability.
- Posterior lumbar tumors.
- Posterior lumbar infection or abscess.

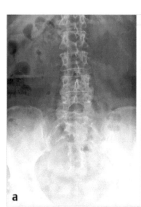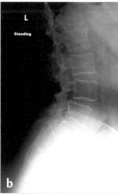

**Fig. 20.1** Anteroposterior **(a)** and lateral **(b)** radiographs. There is a grade 1 degenerative spondylolisthesis at the L4–L5 disk level with spinal stenosis and neuroforaminal narrowing.

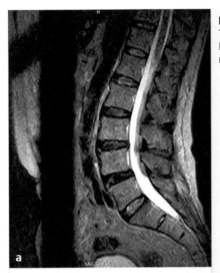

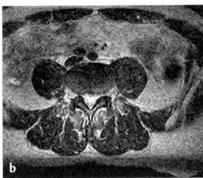

**Fig. 20.2** Sagittal **(a)** and axial **(b)** cuts of a T2-weighted lumbar MRI. There is a grade 1 L4–L5 degenerative spondylolisthesis with moderate spinal stenosis.

## 20.3 Positioning

- Prone position.
- Superficial landmarks include the following:
  - Iliac crest:
    - Typically lies at the L4–L5 intervertebral disk level.
  - Spinous processes:
    - The ideal method of identifying the level of interest is to insert a needle into the spinous process and obtain a radiograph via fluoroscopy.

## 20.4 Approach

- Superficial dissection:
  - Skin incision is made midline at the desired level.
  - The fascia is identified and opened in the midline over the spinous process.

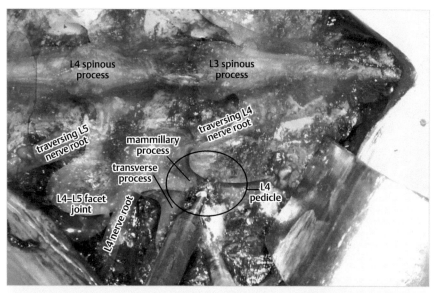

**Fig. 20.3** The pedicle start points are located at the mammillary process at the junction of the inferolateral corner of the facet joint. (Reproduced with permission from Singh K, Vaccaro AR, eds. Pocket Atlas of Spine Surgery. 2nd ed. New York, NY: Thieme; 2018.)

- Subperiosteal dissection of the lumbar paraspinal musculature is performed, exposing the facet joints:
  - ◦ The internervous place is located along the line of incision between the left and right paraspinal muscles:
    - ▪ The lumbar dorsal primary rami supply these muscles.
- Deep dissection:
  - The facet joint is resected and the superior articular process and transverse process of the caudad vertebrae are exposed (**Fig. 20.3**).
  - The pedicle screw starting point is located:
    - ◦ Indicated by the mammillary process:
      - ▪ Junction of the transverse process, lateral pars interarticularis, and super facet.

## 20.5 Implants and Hardware

- The pedicle is tapped and measured:
  - The pedicle screw trajectory ranges from 5 to 20 degrees medially (depending on the lumbar level), increasing with caudal progression.
- Once the pedicle track has been created, it is important to confirm a complete intraosseous trajectory by pedicle and body palpation using a pedicle-sounding device:
  - Subsequent fluoroscopic imaging may be used for confirmation of proper trajectory.
- An appropriate diameter and length screw is inserted (**Fig. 20.4**).

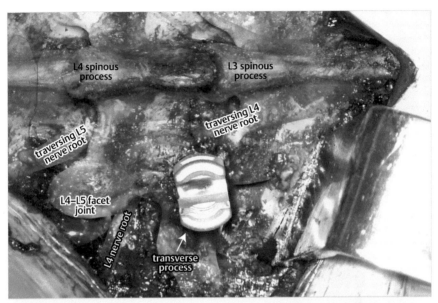

**Fig. 20.4** Posterior view. The pedicle screw has been placed within the boundaries of the pedicle wall. Note the medial and slightly caudal trajectory. (Reproduced with permission from Singh K, Vaccaro AR, eds. Pocket Atlas of Spine Surgery. 2nd ed.  New York, NY: Thieme; 2018.)

• This is repeated for each desired level.
• Rods are inserted to connect the screws.

# 20.6 Case Presentation: Postoperative Outcomes and Imaging

The patient underwent a L4–L5 PLF with placement of unilateral pedicle screws at the right L4 and L5 pedicles. At 6-month follow-up, the patient reports resolution of her radiculopathy with improved strength and sensation. The patient also notes improvement in her low back pain. Postoperative imaging demonstrates stable posterior instrumentation with no evidence of screw loosening or cutout (**Fig. 20.5**).

# 20.7 Complications

• Screw misplacement:
  - Screw positioning beyond the pedicle, resulting in injury to nearby structures:
    ◦ Incidence of approximately 5%.
    ◦ Presents with possible back pain, neurologic dysfunction, dural tears, vascular injury, visceral injury, and/or loss of long-term spinal fixation.

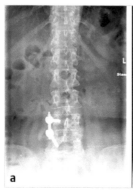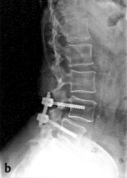

**Fig. 20.5** Anteroposterior **(a)** and lateral **(b)** radiographs. Six-month postoperative radiographs following L4–L5 posterolateral lumbar fusion (PLF) demonstrating appropriate positioning and fixation of unilateral pedicle screws.

- Prevention:
  - Maximize exposure size by performing laminectomy or facetectomy.
  - Utilize preoperative imaging to select for appropriately sized implant based on patient's pedicle width and angulation.
  - Confirm screw placement with intraoperative fluoroscopy.
- Pedicle fracture:
  - Fracture of the lateral wall during pedicle screw placement:
    - Prevents proper anchoring of pedicle screw for appropriate fixation.
  - Risk factors:
    - Osteoporosis.
    - Female sex.
    - Smoking.

## Suggested Readings

1. Inoue M, Inoue G, Ozawa T, et al. L5 spinal nerve injury caused by misplacement of outwardly-inserted S1 pedicle screws. Eur Spine J 2013;22(Suppl 3):S461–S465
2. Esses SI, Sachs BL, Dreyzin V. Complications associated with the technique of pedicle screw fixation. A selected survey of ABS members. Spine 1993;18(15):2231–2238, discussion 2238–2239
3. Amato V, Giannachi L, Irace C, Corona C. Accuracy of pedicle screw placement in the lumbosacral spine using conventional technique: computed tomography postoperative assessment in 102 consecutive patients. J Neurosurg Spine 2010;12(3):306–313
4. Lattig F, Fekete TF, Jeszenszky D. Management of fractures of the pedicle after instrumentation with transpedicular screws: a report of three patients. J Bone Joint Surg Br 2010;92(1):98–102

# 21 Anterior Lumbar Interbody Fusion

*Ankur S. Narain, Fady Y. Hijji, Philip K. Louie, Daniel D. Bohl, and Kern Singh*

## 21.1 Case Presentation and Preoperative Imaging

A 35-year-old woman presents to the office with long-standing axial low back pain. The pain radiates to the bilateral lower extremities, including the right posterior thigh, right lateral calf, and left posterior thigh. Pain is persistent at baseline, but worsens with ambulation and changes in temperature. She denies any trauma or recent infections. Conservative therapy with physical therapy, narcotics, and muscle relaxants provided minimal pain relief. Lumbar magnetic resonance imaging (MRI) was obtained (**Fig. 21.1**).

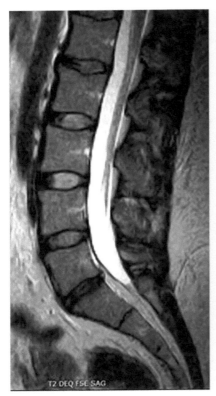

**Fig. 21.1** Sagittal T2-weighted MRI demonstrating L5–S1 retrolisthesis with disk space collapse, central disk protrusion, and a posterior annular tear.

## 21.2 Indications

- Spondylolisthesis (grade I or II).
- Degenerative disk disease.
- Postdiskectomy collapse with neuroforaminal stenosis.
- Revision of posterior pseudoarthrosis or postlaminectomy kyphosis.
- Coronal and/or sagittal imbalance.

## 21.3 Position

- Supine.
- Landmarks:
  - Umbilicus: opposite the L3–L4 disk space.
  - Pubic symphysis: pubic tubercle is located lateral to the midline.

## 21.4 Approach

- Superficial dissection:
  - Skin incision is midline, located between the umbilicus and pubic symphysis (**Fig. 21.2**):
    - The internervous plane is in the midline, as the abdominal musculature is innervated segmentally by the 7th to 12th intercostal nerves.
  - Musculus rectus abdominis fascia incised and the muscle belly is mobilized.
  - The rectus sheath is then incised → exposes the retroperitoneum.

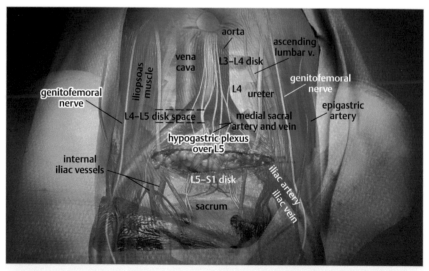

**Fig. 21.2** Top-down view. Skin incision with depiction of underlying anatomic structures. (Reproduced with permission from Singh K, Vaccaro AR, eds. Pocket Atlas of Spine Surgery. 2nd ed. New York, NY: Thieme; 2018).

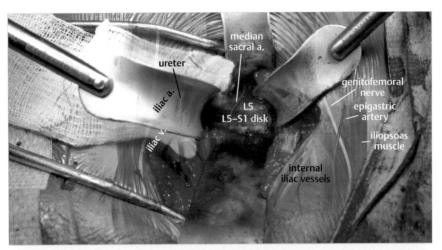

**Fig. 21.3** Top-down view. Deep dissection showing placement of retractors and exposure of the L5–S1 disk in relation to important anatomic landmarks. (Reproduced with permission from Singh K, Vaccaro AR, eds. Pocket Atlas of Spine Surgery. 2nd ed. New York, NY: Thieme; 2018.)

- Deep dissection:
  - Retroperitoneum is swept laterally and retractors are placed when the psoas is encountered (**Fig. 21.3**):
    ○ Care must be taken to avoid nerve injury to the adjacent presacral plexus or iliolumbar artery, depending on level of pathology.
    ○ Identify and ligate the middle sacral artery to prevent hemorrhage.
    ○ Visceral injury to the great vessels or ureters can occur. Identify and retract these structures out of the operative field.
  - Soft tissues in front of the disk space are retracted medially.
  - Bluntly dissect and clear off the disk space.
  - Perform annulotomy and remove disk fragments.
  - Prepare end plates.

## 21.5 Hardware and Implants

- After sequential distraction of the end plates, continue diskectomy posteriorly until the posterior annulus is visualized.
- Clear foramen laterally via microcurette.
- Interbody cages filled with autologous or allograft bone are placed with screw fixation into the cephalad and caudad vertebral bodies.

## 21.6 Case Presentation: Postoperative Imaging and Outcome

The patient underwent an anterior lumbar interbody fusion (ALIF) with placement of a stand-alone interbody cage. She experienced significant improvement in

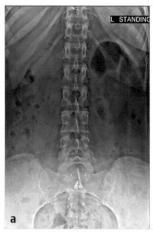 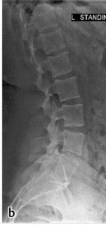

**Fig. 21.4** Anteroposterior **(a)** and lateral **(b)** plain radiographs demonstrating adequate placement of the interbody cage with screw fixation. Good bony consolidation is seen.

pain at 6 months postoperatively. Good bony consolidation was demonstrated on postoperative imaging studies (**Fig. 21.4**).

## 21.7 Complications

- Presacral plexus injury:
  - Caused by manipulation of the plexus during dissection.
  - Presents with retrograde ejaculation ± impotence.
  - Prevention:
    ∘ Ensure midline incision is long enough for nerve mobilization.
    ∘ Avoid use of monopolar cautery.
- Great vessel injury:
  - Due to improper retraction during exposure.
  - Presents with hemorrhage; can be fatal.
  - Prevention:
    ∘ Ligation of penetrating lumbar vessels allows for more effective retraction of great vessels.
  - Treatment:
    ∘ Hemostasis, primary suture or double ligature repair.
    ∘ Vascular surgery consultation.
- Abdominal complications:
  - Ileus:
    ∘ Presents with abdominal distention, discomfort, decreased flatulence.
    ∘ Treatment:
      ▪ Place patient NPO (nil per os), administer intravenous (IV) fluids, and bowel rest.
      ▪ Laxatives and slow advancement of diet as symptoms resolve.
  - Ureteral injury:
    ∘ Occurs during deep dissection adjacent to the disk space.
    ∘ Prevention:
      ▪ Identification within the surgical field and lateral retraction.

- Subsidence, end plate fracture, graft dislodgement:
  - Caused by improper cage placement and sizing.
  - Presents with retropulsion or pseudoarthrosis on imaging, neuroforaminal impingement leading to focal neurologic deficits.
  - Prevention:
    - Optimizing surgical approach via adequate preoperative imaging.
    - Maintenance of correct surgical orientation via intraoperative fluoroscopy.
    - Testing implant sizes intraoperatively.

## Suggested Readings

1. Sasso RC, Kenneth Burkus J, LeHuec JC. Retrograde ejaculation after anterior lumbar interbody fusion: transperitoneal versus retroperitoneal exposure. Spine 2003;28(10):1023–1026
2. Than KD, Wang AC, Rahman SU, et al. Complication avoidance and management in anterior lumbar interbody fusion. Neurosurg Focus 2011;31(4):E6
3. Tiusanen H, Seitsalo S, Osterman K, Soini J. Retrograde ejaculation after anterior interbody lumbar fusion. Eur Spine J 1995;4(6):339–342

# 22 Minimally Invasive Transforaminal Lumbar Interbody Fusion

*Ankur S. Narain, Fady Y. Hijji, Philip K. Louie, Daniel D. Bohl, and Kern Singh*

## 22.1 Case Presentation

A 52-year-old woman presents to the clinic with right leg pain of 6-month duration. The patient denies any benefit from nonoperative management prescribed by her primary care physician, which included nonsteroidal anti-inflammatory drugs (NSAIDs), epidural steroid injections, and physical therapy. On physical examination, the patient exhibits a positive straight leg test and sensory deficits along the lateral leg. The patient also demonstrates mild weakness on great toe dorsiflexion. There is no noted hypo- or hyperreflexia or Babinski's sign present. Lumbar radiographs are shown in **Figs. 22.1** and **22.2**. The patient's radiographs and magnetic resonance imaging (MRI) are presented. The patient is subsequently scheduled to receive a minimally invasive transforaminal lumbar interbody fusion (MIS TLIF) of the L5S1 disk space.

## 22.2 Indications

- Lumbar disk herniations.
- Compression of lumbar nerve roots.
- Lumbar instability.
- Access to the posterior lumbar spine with minimal blood loss and shortened patient recovery time.

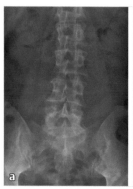 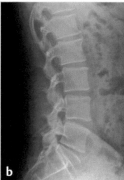

**Fig. 22.1** Anteroposterior **(a)** and lateral **(b)** lumbar radiographs. There is moderate spondylosis of the L5–S1 disk space. Note the loss of disk height and narrowing of the neuroforamen.

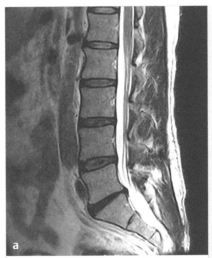

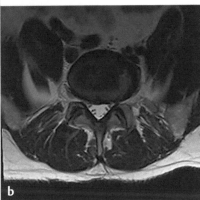

**Fig. 22.2** Sagittal **(a)** and axial **(b)** T2-weighted MRI. There is significant foraminal and moderate central stenosis at the L5–S1 disk level.

## 22.3 Positioning

- Prone.
- Landmarks identified through fluoroscopic imaging:
  - Spinous processes.
  - Pedicular line (lateral edge of the pedicle).

## 22.4 Approach

- Superficial dissection:
  - The skin incision is made lateral to the midpedicular line (1.0 cm; **Fig. 22.3a**):
    - Lateral fluoroscopy is utilized to confirm the location of the placed dilators at the correct level (**Fig. 22.3b**).
    - There is no true internervous plane here, as the incision and entry point is made in between the paraspinal muscles, which are segmentally innervated.

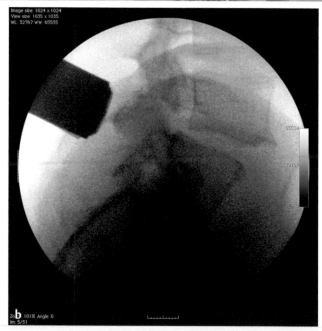

**Fig. 22.3** Intraoperative fluoroscopy showing the placement of a dilator overlying the lamina of the targeted disk level **(a)** with corresponding lateral radiograph **(b)**. Note the off-midline approach. (Reproduced with permission from Singh K, Vaccaro AR, eds. Pocket Atlas of Spine Surgery. 2nd ed. New York, NY: Thieme; 2018.)

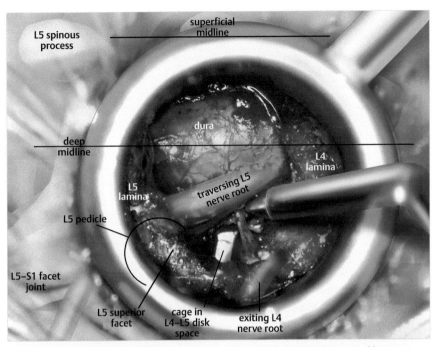

**Fig. 22.4** Top-down view. The lamina, superior and inferior articular facets, and ligamentum flavum have been resected, exposing the dura and nerve root. (Reproduced with permission from Singh K, Vaccaro AR, eds. Pocket Atlas of Spine Surgery. 2nd ed. New York, NY: Thieme; 2018.)

- Dilators are docked over the lamina at the level of pathology with removal of residual paraspinal musculature.
- Deep dissection:
  - The lamina and facet joint are resected:
    - The superior articular process of the caudal vertebrae is removed first during the facetectomy:
      - Inadequate facet removal can result in a narrowed working space, increasing the risk for excessive nerve root retraction and interbody cage misplacement/migration.
  - Once laminectomy and facetectomy are completed, the ligamentum flavum is removed:
    - The disk space, dura, and nerve root are exposed (**Fig. 22.4**).
    - Veins overlying the disk space and dura can cause profuse bleeding.

## 22.5 Implants and Hardware

- The disk space is prepared and cage is impacted into place (**Fig. 22.5**):
  - Complete intervertebral disk removal and appropriate end plate preparation reduces the risk of pseudarthrosis or nonunion.
- Fixation using posterior pedicle screws can be performed from a posterior approach.

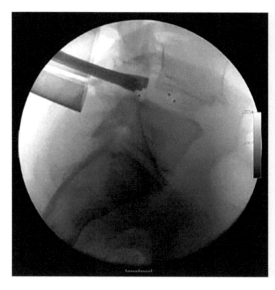

**Fig. 22.5** Intraoperative fluoroscopy shooing the impaction of the interbody device into disk space following complete disk removal and end plate preparation.

## 22.6 Case Presentation: Postoperative Outcome and Imaging

The patient underwent an L5–S1 MIS TLIF with placement of an interbody cage with supplemental fixation using bilateral pedicle screws. At 3-month follow-up, the patient reports resolution of her radiculopathy with improved strength and sensation. The patient also notes minimal low back pain. Postoperative imaging demonstrates stable posterior instrumentation with no evidence of cage migration or pseudoarthrosis (**Figs. 22.6, 22.7**).

## 22.7 Complications

- Nerve root injury:
  - Direct damage of nerve root during or following procedure.
  - Caused by:
    - Intraoperative manipulation or cage misplacement.
    - Compression from potential epidural hematoma:
      - Most commonly affects the inferior nerve root.
  - Prevention:
    - Identify nerve roots located in the working zone prior to diskectomy.
- Durotomy:
  - Tear of the dura with subsequent cerebrospinal fluid (CSF) leak:
    - Often occurs during decompression or ligamentum flavum resection:
      - Rare due to the minimal dural exposure in this approach.
    - Can present with headaches worsened with head elevation or photophobia.

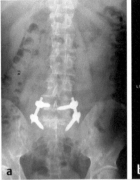
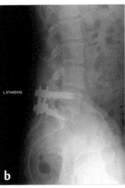

**Fig. 22.6** Anteroposterior **(a)** and lateral **(b)** lumbar radiographs. A 3-month postoperative radiograph following minimally invasive transforaminal lumbar interbody fusion (MIS TLIF) exhibiting placement of an interbody cage with supplemental bilateral fixation.

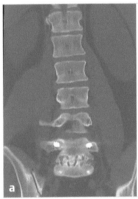
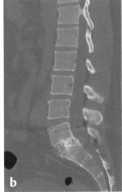

**Fig. 22.7** Postoperative coronal **(a)** and sagittal **(b)** CT scans. Twelve-month postoperative CT scans demonstrating bony bridging at L5–S1 with no evidence of pseudarthrosis.

- Prevention:
  - Refrain from flavum removal until completion of ipsilateral and contralateral neural decompression:
    - Thecal sac protected by dura and pushed ventrally during contralateral decompression.
- Treatment:
  - Primary repair with nonabsorbable sutures.
  - Head elevation during bed rest to reduce pressure on the repair.
- Cage misplacement:
  - Cage migration causing compression of neural structures.
  - Inadequate removal of disk, preparation of vertebral end plates, or damage to anterior longitudinal ligament increase the risk of misplacement.

## Suggested Readings

1.  Wong AP, Smith ZA, Nixon AT, et al. Intraoperative and perioperative complications in minimally invasive transforaminal lumbar interbody fusion: a review of 513 patients. J Neurosurg Spine 2015;22(5):487–495
2.  Knox JB, Dai JM III, Orchowski J. Osteolysis in transforaminal lumbar interbody fusion with bone morphogenetic protein-2. Spine 2011;36(8):672–676

# 23 Lateral Lumbar Interbody Fusion

*Ankur S. Narain, Fady Y. Hijji, Philip K. Louie, Daniel D. Bohl, and Kern Singh*

## 23.1 Case Presentation

A 55-year-old man presents to the clinic complaining of an 8-month history of gradually worsening low back pain. The patient notes bilateral lower extremity radiculopathy radiating to the anteromedial thigh. He has failed multiple trials of physical therapy and steroidal injections. On physical examination, the patient is noted to exhibit a sensory loss on the right anterior thigh. The patient's radiographs and magnetic resonance imaging (MRI) findings are shown in **Figs. 23.1** and **23.2**. The surgeon schedules the patient for a lateral lumbar interbody fusion (LLIF).

## 23.2 Indications

- Lumbar nerve root compression above the level of the iliac crest.
- Lumbar instability.
- Tumors.
- Infection or anterior lumbar abscess.

## 23.3 Positioning

- Lateral decubitus position.
- Superficial landmarks include:
  - Ribs and associated intercostal spaces.
  - Pubic symphysis.
  - Lateral border of rectus abdominis muscle:
    - 5 cm lateral to midline.
  - Spinous processes of desired levels.

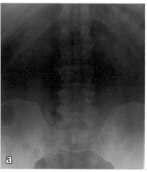 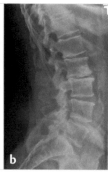

Fig. 23.1 Anteroposterior (a) and lateral (b) lumbar radiographs. Significant spondylosis is apparent at the L2–L3 disk level with radial and anterior osteophyte formation. Note the concurrent retrolisthesis of L2 over L3.

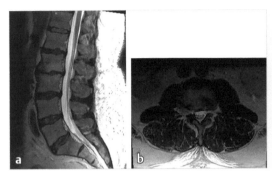

**Fig. 23.2** Sagittal **(a)** and axial **(b)** cuts of a T2-weighted lumbar MRI. There is significant degeneration of the L2–L3 disk with moderate bilateral foraminal stenosis.

# 23.4 Approach

- Superficial dissection:
  - Skin incision made at the lateral aspect of the desired level:
    ○ Fluoroscopy used to determine appropriate level.
  - External oblique, internal oblique, and transversalis fascia are dissected (**Fig. 23.3**):
    ○ No true internervous plane exists in this approach; the muscles of the abdominal wall being divided are segmentally innervated.
- Deep dissection:
  - Transversalis fascia is opened and retroperitoneal fat is exposed and removed.
  - The psoas muscle is then identified and retracted posteriorly or traversed with careful ongoing neuromonitoring (**Fig. 23.4**):
    ○ The lumbar plexus lies within the psoas muscle and can be injured with excessive manipulation.
  - The disk space is identified and prepared.

# 23.5 Implants and Hardware

- The intervertebral disk is completely removed and the end plates are prepared.
- The interbody cage is impacted into the prepared disk space.
- Supplemental percutaneous posterior fixation can be performed using a posterior lumbar approach.

# 23.6 Case Presentation: Postoperative Outcomes and Imaging

The patient underwent an L2–L3 LLIF procedure with placement of an interbody cage and supplemental fixation using unilateral pedicle screws. Postoperatively, the patient complained of new-onset hip flexion weakness with continuing sensory loss of the anterior thigh. However, at his 3-month visit, the patient noted complete resolution of his motor weakness and sensory loss. At his 9-month follow-up, the patient notes

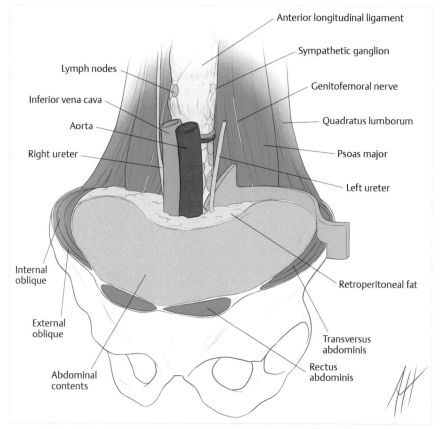

**Fig. 23.3** Lateral view of approach. (Reproduced with permission from Singh K, Vaccaro AR, eds. Pocket Atlas of Spine Surgery. 2nd ed. New York, NY: Thieme; 2018.)

improved lower back pain and no new onset of neurologic symptoms. Postoperative radiographs are presented in **Fig. 23.5**.

# 23.7 Complications

- Visceral or vascular injury:
  - Injury to the bowels, great vessels, and ureters can occur during exposure and retraction of abdominal contents:
    - Visceral injury can present with peritonitis and abdominal pain.
    - Vascular injury can present with hemorrhage, hypotension, and/or progressive neurologic deficit from expanding hematoma.

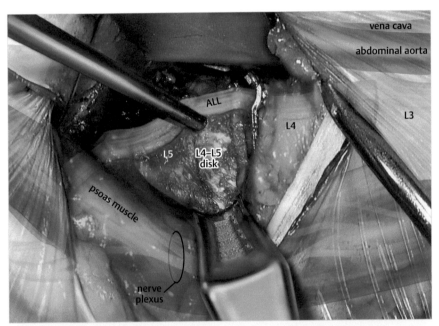

**Fig. 23.4** Top-down view. The psoas muscle and abdominal contents are retracted, exposing the targeted disk space. Note the location of the lumbar plexus within the psoas muscle. (Reproduced with permission from Singh K, Vaccaro AR, eds. Pocket Atlas of Spine Surgery. 2nd ed. New York, NY: Thieme; 2018.)

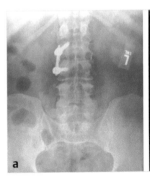 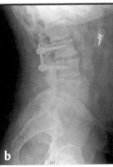

**Fig. 23.5** Anteroposterior **(a)** and lateral **(b)** views. A 9-month postoperative radiograph following lateral lumbar interbody fusion (LLIF) showing placement of an interbody cage at L2–L3 with supplemental unilateral pedicle screw fixation.

- Prevention:
  - Meticulous finger dissection to palpate visceral structures prior to retractor placement.
  - Sweep all structures posteriorly, protected by the dilators or retractors.
- Neural injury:
  - Injury to the lumbosacral plexus or sympathetic ganglion during exposure and psoas retraction:

- ◦ Thigh weakness, pain, and sensory loss.
- ◦ Transient sensory loss and hip flexion weakness are extremely common following LLIF and usually resolve within 4 to 6 weeks:
  - ▪ Attributed to psoas trauma rather than true neurologic injury.
- – Prevention:
  - ◦ Neuromonitoring to identify potential injury to lumbar plexus.
  - ◦ Intermittent relaxation of muscle retraction, especially during multilevel or prolonged cases.

## Suggested Readings

1. Grimm BD, Leas DP, Poletti SC, Johnson DR II. Postoperative complications within the first year after extreme lateral interbody fusion: experience of the first 108 patients. Clin Spine Surg 2016;29(3):E151–E156

2. Härtl R, Joeris A, McGuire RA. Comparison of the safety outcomes between two surgical approaches for anterior lumbar fusion surgery: anterior lumbar interbody fusion (ALIF) and extreme lateral interbody fusion (ELIF). Eur Spine J 2016;25(5):1484–1521

# 24 Surgical Complications

*Ikechukwu Achebe, Ankur S. Narain, Fady Y. Hijji, Philip K. Louie, Daniel D. Bohl, and Kern Singh*

## 24.1 Introduction

Surgery is inherently associated with risk. Surgeries involving the spine and spinal cord are subject to various severe complications, and thus warrant additional intervention. An understanding of these complications, along with appropriate prevention and treatment strategies, is essential to patient safety. Therefore, it is important to recognize the etiology, presentation, and management strategies for common surgical complications including postoperative fever, surgical site infection, durotomy, and spinal epidural hematoma (**Table 24.1**).

**Table 24.1** Common etiologies of postoperative fever

| Etiology | Approximate day of onset | Clinical evaluation | Imaging | Primary treatment |
|---|---|---|---|---|
| Surgical trauma and tissue manipulation | POD 0 | – | – | Self-limited |
| Atelectasis | POD 1–2 | Incentive spirometry | CXR | Oxygen therapy Pulmonary rehabilitation |
| Pneumonia | POD 3 | WBC, sputum culture | CXR | Antibiotics Pulmonary therapy |
| UTI | POD 2–3 | Urinalysis, urine culture | – | Antibiotics Catheter removal or replacement |
| DVT/PE | POD 3–7 | D-dimer | CT angiogram, duplex ultrasonography | Anticoagulation |
| Wound infection or bacteremia | POD 3–7 | WBC, ESR, CRP, blood culture, wound culture | MRI | Antibiotics Wound care Debridement and removal of hardware |
| Implant infection | Delayed (weeks to months) | ESR, CRP, WBC, wound culture | MRI | Antibiotics Debridement Hardware removal |

Abbreviations: CRP, C-reactive protein; CT, computed tomography; CXR, chest X-ray; DVT, deep vein thrombosis; ESR, erythrocyte sedimentation rate; MRI, magnetic resonance imaging; PE, pulmonary embolism; POD, postoperative day; UTI, urinary tract infection; WBC, white blood cell.

## 24.2 Postoperative Fever

• Background:
  – Body temperature greater than 38.6°C (101.5°F).
  – Incidence rate of 14 to 91%.
• Etiology:
  – Immediate onset:
    ◦ Majority are noninfectious (>50% of cases).
  – Acute, subacute, and delayed onset:
    ◦ Strongly consider infectious etiology.
• Risk factors:
  – Immunosuppression, prolonged operative time, nosocomial infections.
  – Urinary catheterization, respiratory ventilation.
• Presentation:
  – Diaphoresis, chills, headache.

## 24.3 Surgical Site Infections

• Background:
  – Postoperative infection localized to surgical site; occurs within 30 days.
  – Incidence following spine surgery is 1 to 12%.
  – Surgical site infection (SSI) types and associated tissues (Fig. 24.1).
• Etiology:
  – Routes of infection:
    ◦ Direct Inoculation of skin flora.
    ◦ Wound contamination.
  – SSI pathogens association:
    ◦ Gram (+): *Staphylococcus. aureus* (50% of SSIs), *S. epidermidis,* and *Streptococcus.*
    ◦ Gram (–): *Pseudomonas. aeruginosa, Escherichia coli,* and *Proteus.*
• Risk factors:
  – Preoperative: diabetes, smoking history, body mass index (BMI), corticosteroid use, age.
  – Intraoperative: sterile technique, invasiveness, operative duration.
  – SSI risk by procedure: trauma > diskitis > tumor resection > minimally invasive.
  – SSI risk by location: thoracic (2.1%) > lumbar (1.6%) > cervical (0.8%) vertebrae.
• Presentation:
  – Clinical symptoms:
    ◦ Back pain, wound drainage, erythema, palpable fluctuance.
    ◦ Fever, fatigue (deep SSI [DSSI] > SSSI).
• Clinical evaluation:
  – Laboratory tests:
    ◦ Erythrocyte sedimentation rate (ESR), C-reactive protein (CRP) elevation (high sensitivity 94–100%).
    ◦ White blood cell (WBC) elevation (poor sensitivity 44–58%).

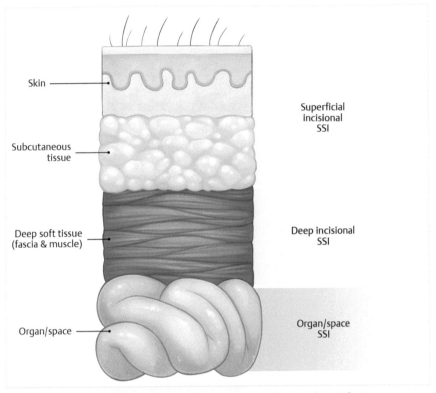

**Fig. 24.1** Centers for Disease Control and Prevention (CDC) surgical site infection classification.

- Bacterial cultures:
  - Positive in 51 and 78% of SSSI and DSSI cases, respectively.
  - Intraoperative and deep cultures preferred.
- Radiographic evaluation:
  - Magnetic resonance imaging (MRI) at 3 to 5 days postoperatively (sensitivity 93%):
    - T2: edema appears as hyperintense signal.
    - Decreased height of vertebral disk/body seen with late stage infection.
  - Radionucleotide imaging: increased uptake of 67Ga at sites of infection.
  - X-ray: decreased intervertebral height discernable 4 to 6 weeks postoperatively.
  - Computed tomography (CT): bony destruction, soft-tissue abscesses.
- Treatment:
  - Antibiotics, wound care:
    - Start antibiotics with broad coverage and narrow upon determination of causative organism.
  - If conservative treatment fails or symptoms progress: debridement, removal of hardware.

# 24.4 Durotomy

- Background:
  - Incidental tear of dura mater.
  - Severity determines need for corrective surgery (1–17% of tears).
  - Cerebrospinal fluid (CSF) leak may create fistulas and pseudomeningoceles.
- Etiology:
  - Direct injury from instrumentation or injection **(Fig. 24.2)**.
  - Failed dural repair (i.e., tumor/cyst resection, shunt placement).
- Risk factors:
  - Preoperative: diabetes, smoking, age, BMI, radiation, or steroid therapy.
  - Intraoperative: procedure invasiveness, revision surgery.
  - Risk by primary diagnosis: spinal trauma (20%) > degenerative stenosis (11.2%) > tumors (10.5%) > lumbar disk herniations (8%).
  - Risk by surgery location: thoracic (2.2%) > lumbar (2.1%) > cervical (1%) spine.
- Cutaneous CSF fistula:
  - Etiology:
    - Residual opening permits leak **(Fig. 24.3)**.
    - CSF drains along surgical tract.
    - Infection can occur (meningitis).

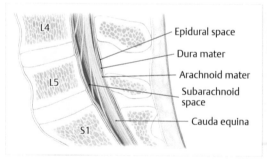

**Fig. 24.2** Vertebrae and their association with the meningeal layers.

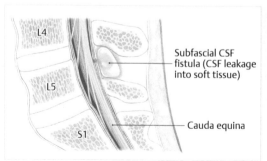

**Fig. 24.3** Cutaneous cerebrospinal fluid (CSF) fistula with leakage into the adjacent soft-tissue space.

- Presentation:
  - Postural headache, CSF discharge, fever, neck stiffness, pain.
- Clinical evaluation:
  - Clear drainage (CSF) at incision site..
  - Valsalva maneuver aggravates CSF leak and headache.
  - Lab tests:
    - Drainage fluids are Beta-2 transferrin positive.
- Imaging:
  - MRI shows T2-hyperintense extra-arachnoid fluid.
- Treatment:
  - Wound suture with optional hemostatic agents.
  - Drainage, epidural blood patch, bed rest.
  - Dural repair surgery:
    - Indications: severe CSF leak.
    - Contraindications: poor CSF absorption, high intradural pressure.
- Pseudomeningocele:
  - Etiology:
    - Arachnoid herniation through dural opening leading to nerve compression.
    - CSF leakage into paraspinal or local tissues contributes to nerve compression **(Fig. 24.4)**.
  - Presentation:
    - Postural headache, swelling, back pain, delayed-onset radiculopathy.
  - Clinical evaluation:
    - Valsalva maneuver leads to aggravation of headache.
  - Imaging:
    - MRI:
      - T1-hypointense mass in the posterior spine.
      - T2-hyperintense cystic CSF-filled mass.

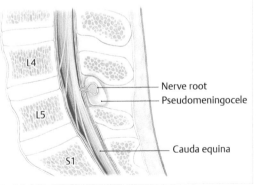

**Fig. 24.4** Pseudomeningocele depicted by an arachnoid herniation leading to nerve root entrapment.

- Treatment:
  - ◦ Drainage (3–5 days).
  - ◦ Epidural blood patch.
  - ◦ Dural repair surgery (nonurgent):
    - ▪ Indications and contraindications similar to that for cutaneous CSF fistula.

# 24.5  Spinal Epidural Hematoma

- Background:
  - Bleeding into the potential space between bone and dura mater **(Fig. 24.5)**:
    - ◦ Symptoms range from asymptomatic to severe neurologic complications due to cord compression.
  - Incidence: 0.1 to 1%.
- Etiology:
  - Spine surgery (iatrogenic).
  - Spinal tap or anesthesia.
- Risk factors:
  - Preoperative: coagulopathy, antithrombotics, higher in females than in males, age older than 60 years.
  - Intraoperative: multilevel procedures, prior surgeries.
- Presentation:
  - Rapid onset and symptom progression:
    - ◦ Bilateral motor and sensory deficits (68% of patients).
    - ◦ Gastrointestinal (GI)/genitourinary (GU) dysfunction (8%).
    - ◦ Severe back pain ± radicular symptoms.
- Radiographic evaluation:
  - MRI: First line:
    - ◦ T1 hypointense and T2 hyperintense in the acute stage.
    - ◦ T1 and T2 hyperintense in the subacute stage.
  - CT ± myelography.

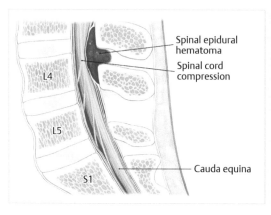

**Fig. 24.5** Spinal epidural hematoma with resultant cord compression.

Spinal epidural hematoma

Spinal cord compression

L4

L5

Cauda equina

S1

- Treatment:
  - Surgical decompression with evacuation.
  - Conservative therapy involves use of intravenous (IV) steroids:
    - Indicated when symptomatology improves prior to potential operative therapy.

# 24.6  Pedicle Screw Misplacement

- Background:
  - Occurs in 7.8% of cases involving pedicle instrumentation.
  - Greater than 4 mm displacement is associated with a high risk of injury to adjacent structures.
- Etiology:
  - Malpositioning of the pedicle secondary to:
    - Guide wire pullout.
    - Improper targeting of pedicular structures.
    - Erosion of metal–bone interface leading to screw displacement.
- Presentation:
  - Varies based on anatomical direction of misplacement:
    - Medial or inferior violation: nerve root or spinal cord injury (0.6–11%).
    - Lateral violation: injuries to aorta, segmental vessels, lung parenchyma, pneumothorax.
    - Anterior violation: injuries to aorta, vena cava, esophagus.
  - Pedicle fracture (1.1%).
  - Screw breakage (3.0–5.7%).
- Radiographic evaluation:
  - Postoperative CT:
    - Axial sections best demonstrate screw position (**Fig. 24.6**):
      - Adjacent areas of radiolucency may indicate improper placement.
    - Can demonstrate pedicle or vertebral body fractures.
- Management:
  - Prevention:
    - Ensure proper guide wire targeting.
    - Ensure adequate preoperative characterization of anatomy and screw sizing via imaging.
    - Screw augmentation via polymethylmethacrylate, hydroxyapatite, calcium phosphate, or carbonated apatite.
    - Use of surgical assistance techniques (intraoperative fluoroscopy, robotic assisted).
  - Treatment:
    - Repair of damaged vasculature or visceral structures.
    - Revision with alternate screw trajectory or extension of fusion.

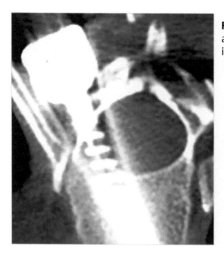

**Fig. 24.6** Axial computed tomography image demonstrating medial pedicle violation into the thecal sac.

## Suggested Readings

1.  Amiri AR, Fouyas IP, Cro S, Casey AT. Postoperative spinal epidural hematoma (SEH): incidence, risk factors, onset, and management. Spine J 2013;13(2):134–140
2.  An HS, Jenis LG. Spinal cord injury, incidental durotomy, and epidural hematoma. In: Complications of Spine Surgery: Treatment and Prevention. Philadelphia, PA: Lippincott Williams & Wilkins; 2006:38–39
3.  Benzel EC, Francis TB, Basheal A, et al. Perioperative management/postoperative complications. In: Spine Surgery: Techniques, Complication Avoidance, and Management. Philadelphia, PA: Elsevier/Saunders; 2012:1727–1742
4.  Benzel EC, Francis TB, Connolly E, Long D. Spine reoperations. In: Varma G, ed. Spine Surgery: Techniques, Complication Avoidance, and Management. Philadelphia, PA: Elsevier/Saunders; 2012:1921–1926
5.  Chahoud J, Kanafani Z, Kanj SS. Surgical site infections following spine surgery: eliminating the controversies in the diagnosis. Front Med (Lausanne) 2014;1:7
6.  Cohn SL, Cooper B. Postoperative fever. In: Fair N, ed. Perioperative Medicine. London: Springer; 2011:411–413
7.  Epstein NE. A review article on the diagnosis and treatment of cerebrospinal fluid fistulas and dural tears occurring during spinal surgery. Surg Neurol Int 2013;4(Suppl 5):S301–S317
8.  Kalevski SK, Peev NA, Haritonov DG. Incidental Dural Tears in lumbar decompressive surgery: incidence, causes, treatment, results. Asian J Neurosurg 2010;5(1):54–59
9.  Kim T, Lee CH, Hyun SJ, Yoon SH, Kim KJ, Kim HJ. Clinical Outcomes of Spontaneous Spinal Epidural Hematoma: A Comparative Study between Conservative and Surgical Treatment. J Korean Neurosurg Soc 2012;52(6):523–527
10. Nam KH, Choi CH, Yang MS, Kang DW. Spinal epidural hematoma after pain control procedure. J Korean Neurosurg Soc 2010;48(3):281–284
11. Pull ter Gunne AF, Mohamed AS, Skolasky RL, van Laarhoven CJ, Cohen DB. The presentation, incidence, etiology, and treatment of surgical site infections after spinal surgery. Spine 2010;35(13):1323–1328

12. Smith JS, Shaffrey CI, Sansur CA, et al; Scoliosis Research Society Morbidity and Mortality Committee. Rates of infection after spine surgery based on 108, 419 procedures: a report from the Scoliosis Research Society Morbidity and Mortality Committee. Spine 2011;36(7):556–563

13. Walid MS, Woodall MN, Nutter JP, Ajjan M, Robinson JS Jr. Causes and risk factors for postoperative fever in spine surgery patients. South Med J 2009;102(3):283–286

14. Williams BJ, Sansur CA, Smith JS, et al. Incidence of unintended durotomy in spine surgery based on 108,478 cases. Neurosurgery 2011;68(1):117–123, discussion 123–124

15. Bydon M, Xu R, Amin AG, et al. Safety and efficacy of pedicle screw placement using intraoperative computed tomography: consecutive series of 1148 pedicle screws. J Neurosurg Spine 2014;21(3):320–328

16. Gautschi OP, Schatlo B, Schaller K, Tessitore E. Clinically relevant complications related to pedicle screw placement in thoracolumbar surgery and their management: a literature review of 35,630 pedicle screws. Neurosurg Focus 2011;31(4):E8

17. Faraj AA, Webb JK. Early complications of spinal pedicle screw. Eur Spine J 1997;6(5):324–326

18. Matsuzaki H, Tokuhashi Y, Matsumoto F, Hoshino M, Kiuchi T, Toriyama S. Problems and solutions of pedicle screw plate fixation of lumbar spine. Spine 1990;15(11):1159–1165

19. O'Brien JR, Krushinski E, Zarro CM, Sciadini M, Gelb D, Ludwig S. Esophageal injury from thoracic pedicle screw placement in a polytrauma patient: a case report and literature review. J Orthop Trauma 2006;20(6):431–434

# 25 Common Medical Complications Following Routine Spinal Surgery

*Ankur S. Narain, Fady Y. Hijji, Benjamin Khechen, Brittany E. Haws, Philip K. Louie, Daniel D. Bohl, and Kern Singh*

## 25.1 Gastrointestinal Complications

### 25.1.1 Postoperative Nausea and Vomiting

- Background and etiology:
  - Incidence rates approach 20 to 30% of patients undergoing spinal procedures.
  - Risk factors include the following:
    - Patient factors: female gender, history of motion sickness or postoperative nausea and vomiting (PONV), nonsmokers, younger age.
    - Surgical factors: extended duration of anesthesia.
    - Pharmacologic factors: postoperative opioids.
- Management:
  - Prevention:
    - Avoid general anesthesia and volatile anesthetics if possible.
    - Limit opioid use.
    - Promote adequate hydration.
  - Treatment:
    - Antiemetics.
      - 5-HT3 receptor antagonists, neurokinin 1 (Nk-1) receptor antagonists, corticosteroids, butyrophenones, antihistamines, anticholinergics, phenothiazines.
      - Use of dopamine and serotonin antagonist medication is associated with QT prolongation; monitoring of echocardiogram (ECG) for QT interval and presence of arrhythmias is recommended.

### 25.1.2 Dysphagia

- Background and etiology:
  - Incidence rate approaching 71% following cervical procedures; most common in the first postoperative week.
  - Risk factors include the following:
    - Patient factors: female gender, older age.
    - Surgical factors: multilevel procedures, revision procedures, procedures involving lower cervical levels (C4–C6).
  - Etiology is multifactorial and may involve manipulation of esophageal tissue during surgery, hardware displacement, esophageal perforation, retropharyngeal abscesses, or neural injury.

- Presentation:
  - Reflexive coughing.
  - Difficulty swallowing food or drink with leakage.
  - Risk for aspiration and possible pneumonia.
- Clinical evaluation:
  - Bedside swallowing test.
  - Speech/language pathology consultation.
- Radiographic evaluation:
  - Cervical radiographs: to evaluate for structural etiologies.
  - Videofluoroscopic/modified barium swallow study: allows for evaluation of the pharynx and esophagus:
    - Soft-tissue swelling with displacement of the esophagus is the most common finding.
    - Can additionally evaluate for hardware failure.
- Management:
  - Prevention:
    - Avoidance of prolonged operative time.
    - Intermittent relaxation of self-retaining retractors and partial deflation of the endotracheal cuff once retractors are in place.
    - Instrumentation modifications (anchored spacer, smaller cervical plates).
  - Treatment:
    - Nothing by mouth (NPO) or restricted dietary status:
      - Consider nasogastric (NG) or percutaneous endoscopic gastrostomy (PEG) tube placement if severe dysfunction with aspiration risk and nutritional deficits is present.
    - Behavioral modifications: postural changes, swallowing maneuvers.

## 25.1.3 Postoperative Ileus

- Background and etiology:
  - Incidence rate of 3.5% after elective spinal procedures (most common after anterior lumbar and lateral retroperitoneal procedures).
  - Risk factors include the following:
    - Patient factors: older age, male gender, previous opioid use, history of gastroesophageal reflux disease (GERD), history of abdominal surgery.
    - Surgical factors: anterior or lateral surgical approaches.
  - Etiology involves failure of peristalsis due to a pathologic response by the gastrointestinal (GI) tract to surgical manipulation and tissue trauma:
    - Underlying sepsis and electrolyte abnormalities (hypokalemia, hyponatremia, and hypomagnesemia) may worsen ileus.
- Presentation:
  - Pain, nausea, vomiting, abdominal distention, inability to pass flatus or stool.
- Radiographic evaluation:
  - Abdominal radiographs:
    - Identify possible bowel distention or transition points indicative of mechanical obstruction.

- Computed tomography (CT) scan:
  - Evaluate for mechanical obstruction or bowel injury.
- Management:
  - Prevention:
    - Limit bowel manipulation.
    - Minimize narcotic consumption.
  - Treatment:
    - Place patient NPO for bowel rest.
    - Administer intravenous (IV) fluids for electrolyte correction.
    - Laxatives and slow diet advancement as tolerated.
    - For patients with vomiting and distention, a nasogastric tube may provide symptomatic relief; however, there is no conclusive evidence that nasogastric tubes facilitate resolution of ileus.

# 25.2 Pulmonary and Respiratory Complications

## 25.2.1 Airway Compromise and Reintubation

- Background and etiology:
  - Incidence approaching 6.1% of patients undergoing cervical spine surgery.
  - Risk factors include the following:
    - Patient factors: morbid obesity, obstructive sleep apnea, history of pulmonary disease, low preoperative hematocrit, high serum creatinine.
    - Surgical factors: exposures involving more than three vertebral bodies, blood loss greater than 300 mL, exposures of C2–C4, operative time greater than 5 hours, anteroposterior approach.
  - Etiologies include laryngopharynx and prevertebral soft-tissue edema, hematoma, cerebrospinal fluid (CSF) leaks, or hardware dislodgement.
    - Presentation after 12 hours postoperatively is associated with airway edema.
    - Delayed presentation after 72 hours postoperatively is associated with hematoma, CSF leaks, hardware failure.
- Presentation:
  - Dyspnea, dysphonia.
  - Can progress to stridor, cyanosis.
  - Increased risk of aspiration.
- Clinical evaluation:
  - Arterial blood gases demonstrate hypercarbia and hypoxia.
- Radiographic evaluation:
  - Plain radiographs and CT scan:
    - Lateral views often demonstrate prevertebral soft-tissue swelling.
- Management:
  - Prevention:
    - In high-risk patients, consider delayed extubation with postoperative intensive care unit (ICU) admission.

- Treatment:
  - Emergent intubation is required if there is evidence of airway compromise.

## 25.2.2 Pneumonia

- Background and etiology:
  - Incidence ranges from 0.45 to 1.05% depending on surgical location.
  - Risk factors include the following:
    - Cervical procedures: Older age, chronic obstructive pulmonary disease (COPD), increased operative time, dependent functional status.
    - Lumbar procedures: COPD, diabetes, increased number of operative levels, steroid use.
  - Etiology is multifactorial:
    - Endotracheal intubation can lead to mini-aspirations.
    - Postoperative atelectasis reduces air movement.
    - Postoperative dysphagia poses an additional aspiration risk.
- Presentation:
  - Fever, dyspnea, productive cough often presenting postoperative day 3 (POD3) or later.
  - Associated with higher rates of sepsis, mortality, and readmission.
- Clinical evaluation:
  - White blood cells (WBCs).
  - Sputum culture.
- Radiographic evaluation:
  - Chest radiography: pattern of infiltrate can help determine etiology:
    - Lobar infiltrates are associated with bacterial sources.
    - Diffuse, interstitial infiltrates are associated with viral sources.
    - Infiltrates in dependent areas are associated with aspiration:
      - If patients are upright: inferior lung segments.
      - If patients are supine: posterior lung segments.
  - CT scan: allows for detailed evaluation:
    - Detection of complications such as pleural effusions or abscess formation.
- Management:
  - Prevention:
    - Elevation of head of bed to 30 degrees and sitting up for all meals to prevent aspiration.
    - Oral hygiene.
    - Pulmonary rehabilitation with incentive spirometry to prevent atelectasis.
    - Adequate analgesia.
    - Supervised ambulation.
  - Treatment:
    - Antibiotics.
    - Pulmonary rehabilitation.

# 25.3 Cardiac Complications

## 25.3.1 Myocardial Infarction

• Background and etiology:
  - Incidence ranges from 1 to 2% after spinal procedures.
  - Risk factors include the following:
    ◦ Patient factors: older age (>65 years), atrial fibrillation, hypertension, prior MI, current anticoagulation requirement.
    ◦ Abnormal lab values: low albumin, creatinine greater than 1 mg/dL.
    ◦ Surgical factors: traumatic indication, two-level fusion, intraoperative transfusion requirement, length of stay greater than 7 days.
  - Etiology:
    ◦ Associated with decreased coronary perfusion secondary to operative blood loss.
    ◦ Hypotension and hemodynamic instability are also more frequent in the prone position due to decreases in blood pressure and cardiac function.
• Presentation:
  - Crushing chest pain with radiation to the shoulder, arm, and jaw.
  - Dyspnea, diaphoresis.
• Clinical evaluation:
  - ECG changes differ by type and location of MI:
    ◦ Non-ST–segment elevation MI (NSTEMI): ST-segment flattening, T-wave flattening or inversion.
    ◦ ST-segment elevation MI (STEMI): ST elevation in ischemic areas, ST depression in reciprocal areas, Q-wave formation.
    ◦ Troponin and creatine kinase-MB (CK-MB) levels:
      ▪ Elevated in both STEMI and NSTEMI.
  - Radiographic evaluation:
    ◦ ECG can be used to detect wall motion abnormalities:
      ▪ Do not delay treatment for radiographic examinations if there is significant clinical suspicion for MI.
  - Management:
    ◦ All patients receive morphine for pain control, supplemental oxygen, nitrates, aspirin, beta-blockers, and statins.
    ◦ STEMI: emergent percutaneous revascularization or fibrinolytic therapy.
    ◦ NSTEMI: anticoagulation, possible escalation to revascularization therapy based on cardiac catheterization findings.

## 25.3.2 Stroke and Cerebrovascular Accident

• Background and etiology:
  - Incidence rates approximately 0.22% after spine surgery.
  - Risk factors include the following:

- Patient factors: older age, greater comorbidity burden.
- Surgical factors: cervical procedures, spinal cord tumor resection, increased length of stay.
  - Etiology:
    - Can be either ischemic (most common) or hemorrhagic:
      - Hypothesized to involve increasing rates of intracranial hemorrhage secondary to postoperative CSF leak.

• Presentation:
  - Most common symptoms include dysarthria, hemiparesis.
  - Other symptoms include weakness, numbness, headache, nonorthostatic dizziness.

• Clinical evaluation:
  - Neurology consultation.
  - Imperative to determine time of symptom onset.
  - National Institutes of Health (NIH) stroke scale:
    - 42-point scale, higher scores indicate increased likelihood for stroke.

• Radiographic evaluation:
  - CT without contrast:
    - Evaluates for presence of hemorrhage.
    - Can be performed quickly and is sufficient in most emergency cases.
  - Magnetic resonance imaging (MRI): more sensitive than CT.
    - Significant time requirement compared to CT.
    - Contraindicated in those with contrast allergy, presence of instrumentation.
  - Computed tomography angiography (CTA) or magnetic resonance angiography (MRA):
    - Indicated when possible endovascular procedures are planned.

• Management:
  - Ischemic stroke:
    - Recombinant tissue plasminogen activator (rTPA) if presenting within 3 to 4.5 hours of symptom onset.
    - Can also consider intra-arterial thrombolysis or endovascular techniques up to 6 hours from symptom onset.
    - After therapy: patients are placed on antiplatelet medications, anticoagulants, and blood pressure control.
  - Hemorrhagic stroke
    - Blood pressure and intracranial pressure monitoring.
    - Discontinuing anticoagulant medications.
    - Consult neurosurgery for possible surgical decompression:
      - Indicated if the following sources of bleeding are identified:
        ❖ Aneurysm.
        ❖ Arteriovenous malformation.
        ❖ High intracranial pressure.

# 25.4 Urinary Complications

## 25.4.1 Postoperative Urinary Retention

- Background and etiology:
  - Reported incidence of 5.6 to 38% following spine procedures.
  - Risk factors:
    - Patient factors: older age, male gender, history of benign prostatic hypertrophy, diabetes, depression, myelopathy.
    - Surgical factors: intraoperative Foley catheterization.
    - Pharmacological factors: administration of phenylephrine or neostigmine.
- Presentation:
  - Bladder or abdominal distention.
  - Suprapubic tenderness.
  - Inability to void despite sensation of a full bladder.
- Evaluation:
  - Necessity for catheterization indicates increased likelihood of retention.
  - Blood urea nitrogen (BUN), creatinine levels.
  - Urinalysis.
  - Consider digital rectal examination if concerned for cauda equina syndrome.
- Radiographic evaluation:
  - Bladder ultrasonography can determine postvoid residuals.
- Management:
  - Prevention:
    - Avoid excessive opioid use:
      - Multimodal analgesia has been associated with decreased rates of postoperative urinary retention (POUR).
    - Limiting postoperative indwelling catheter time.
  - Treatment:
    - Intermittent catheterization: majority of patients have self-limited symptomatology after evacuation of residual urine:
      - Urethral catheterization.
      - Suprapubic catheterization.
    - Alpha-adrenergic medications.
    - Cholinergic medications.

## 25.4.2 Urinary Tract Infection

- Background and etiology:
  - 2-3% incidence after spinal procedures.
  - Risk factors include the following:
    - Patient factors: increased comorbidity burden, elevated postoperative C-reactive protein (CRP), older age, female gender, creatinine greater than 1.5 mg/dL.
    - Surgical factors: increased operative time.

- Etiology:
  - ◦ Interference of normal voiding, presence of indwelling catheters, introduction of bacteria in a nosocomial setting.
- Presentation:
  - Dysuria, urgency, frequency, suprapubic pain, hematuria.
  - Assess for flank pain and costovertebral angle (CVA) tenderness.

- Clinical evaluation
  - Urinalysis.
  - Urine culture with susceptibilities.

- Radiographic evaluation:
  - CT scan: used to identify pyelonephritis or abscesses.
    - ◦ Indicated if there is evidence of pyelonephritis such as fever, flank pain, CVA tenderness.

- Treatment:
  - Antibiotics: fluoroquinolones with renal clearance:
    - ◦ Narrow spectrum upon identification of organism and susceptibilities.
  - Removal possible sources of infection:
    - ◦ IV catheters, indwelling urinary catheters.

# 25.5 Vascular and Hematologic Complications

## 25.5.1 Deep Vein Thrombosis, Venous Thromboembolism, and Pulmonary Embolism

- Background and etiology:
  - Reported incidences following spine procedures.
  - Venous thromboembolism (VTE): 0.3 to 31%:
    - ◦ Pulmonary embolism (PE): 0.3 to 0.4%.
    - ◦ Most cases are diagnosed during the first 2 postoperative weeks.
  - Risk factors include the following:
    - ◦ Patient factors: body mass index (BMI) > 40 kg/m2, older age (>80 years), increased comorbidity burden (American Society of Anesthesiologists [ASA] score > 3), history of VTE, history of factor V Leiden, male sex (PE only).
    - ◦ Surgical factors: prolonged operative time, use of general anesthesia.
  - Etiology:
    - ◦ Combination of postoperative recumbency, venous stasis due to impaired mobility, and hypercoagulable state due to surgical tissue manipulation and local inflammatory response.
- Presentation:
  - Deep vein thrombosis (DVT):
    - ◦ Leg swelling, unilateral leg tenderness.
  - PE:
    - ◦ Dyspnea, tachypnea, pleuritic chest pain, cough, hemoptysis, fever.

- Clinical and radiographic evaluation:
  - DVT:
    - Dependent on risk stratification:
      - Intermediate to high risk:
        - Compression ultrasonography.
      - Low risk:
        - D-dimer: if positive, compression ultrasonography is performed for confirmation.
  - PE:
    - Dependent on risk stratification:
      - High risk:
        - CT pulmonary angiography to detect location of thrombus.
        - Ventilation/perfusion (V/Q) scan to detect areas of mismatch if CT is contraindicated.
      - Low to intermediate risk:
        - D-dimer: if elevated consider further investigation with CT pulmonary angiography or venous duplex ultrasonography for confirmation.
- Management:
  - DVT:
    - Anticoagulation with early ambulation:
      - Must consider postoperative status and invasiveness of recent spine procedure.
    - Consider thrombolytic therapy if the presentation is consistent with impending gangrene.
  - PE:
    - Suspected or confirmed PE with no evidence of shock: anticoagulation.
    - Suspected or confirmed PE with evidence of shock: thrombolysis and anticoagulation.
    - Consider inferior vena cava (IVC) filter if patient has a contraindication to anticoagulation or has recurrent PE on anticoagulation therapy.

## Suggested Readings

1.  Al Maaieh MA, Du JY, Aichmair A, et al. Multivariate analysis on risk factors for postoperative ileus after lateral lumbar interbody fusion. Spine 2014;39(8):688–694
2.  Amsterdam EA, Wenger NK, Brindis RG, et al; American College of Cardiology; American Heart Association Task Force on Practice Guidelines; Society for Cardiovascular Angiography and Interventions; Society of Thoracic Surgeons; American Association for Clinical Chemistry. 2014 AHA/ACC Guideline for the Management of Patients with Non-ST-Elevation Acute Coronary Syndromes: a report of the American College of Cardiology/American Heart Association Task Force on Practice Guidelines. J Am Coll Cardiol 2014;64(24):e139–e228
3.  Anderson KK, Arnold PM. Oropharyngeal Dysphagia after anterior cervical spine surgery: a review. Global Spine J 2013;3(4):273–286

4. Apfel CC, Läärä E, Koivuranta M, Greim CA, Roewer N. A simplified risk score for predicting postoperative nausea and vomiting: conclusions from cross-validations between two centers. Anesthesiology 1999;91(3):693–700
5. Baldini G, Bagry H, Aprikian A, Carli F. Postoperative urinary retention: anesthetic and perioperative considerations. Anesthesiology 2009;110(5):1139–1157
6. Bekelis K, Desai A, Bakhoum SF, Missios S. A predictive model of complications after spine surgery: the National Surgical Quality Improvement Program (NSQIP) 2005-2010. Spine J 2014;14(7):1247–1255
7. Bohl DD, Ahn J, Rossi VJ, Tabaraee E, Grauer JN, Singh K. Incidence and risk factors for pneumonia following anterior cervical decompression and fusion procedures: an ACS-NSQIP study. Spine J 2016;16(3):335–342
8. Bohl DD, Mayo BC, Massel DH, et al. incidence and risk factors for pneumonia after posterior lumbar fusion procedures: an ACS-NSQIP study. Spine 2016;41(12):1058–1063
9. Bohl DD, Webb ML, Lukasiewicz AM, et al. Timing of complications after spinal fusion surgery. Spine 2015;40(19):1527–1535
10. Boulis NM, Mian FS, Rodriguez D, Cho E, Hoff JT. Urinary retention following routine neurosurgical spine procedures. Surg Neurol 2001;55(1):23–27, discussion 27–28
11. Bragg D, El-Sharkawy AM, Psaltis E, Maxwell-Armstrong CA, Lobo DN. Postoperative ileus: Recent developments in pathophysiology and management. Clin Nutr 2015;34(3):367–376
12. Carabini LM, Zeeni C, Moreland NC, et al. Predicting major adverse cardiac events in spine fusion patients: is the revised cardiac risk index sufficient? Spine 2014;39(17):1441–1448
13. Carucci LR, Turner MA, Yeatman CF. Dysphagia secondary to anterior cervical fusion: radiologic evaluation and findings in 74 patients. AJR Am J Roentgenol 2015;204(4):768–775
14. Charen DA, Qian ET, Hutzler LH, Bosco JA. Risk factors for postoperative venous thromboembolism in orthopaedic spine surgery, hip arthroplasty, and knee arthroplasty patients. Bull Hosp Jt Dis (2013) 2015;73(3):198–203
15. Chen CJ, Saulle D, Fu KM, Smith JS, Shaffrey CI. Dysphagia following combined anterior-posterior cervical spine surgeries. J Neurosurg Spine 2013;19(3):279–287
16. Cox JB, Weaver KJ, Neal DW, Jacob RP, Hoh DJ. Decreased incidence of venous thromboembolism after spine surgery with early multimodal prophylaxis: clinical article. J Neurosurg Spine 2014;21(4):677–684
17. Dharmavaram S, Jellish WS, Nockels RP, et al. Effect of prone positioning systems on hemodynamic and cardiac function during lumbar spine surgery: an echocardiographic study. Spine 2006;31(12):1388–1393, discussion 1394
18. Gan TJ, Diemunsch P, Habib AS, et al; Society for Ambulatory Anesthesia. Consensus guidelines for the management of postoperative nausea and vomiting. Anesth Analg 2014;118(1):85–113
19. Gandhi SD, Patel SA, Maltenfort M, et al. Patient and surgical factors associated with postoperative urinary retention after lumbar spine surgery. Spine 2014;39(22):1905–1909
20. Glotzbecker MP, Bono CM, Wood KB, Harris MB. Thromboembolic disease in spinal surgery: a systematic review. Spine 2009;34(3):291–303

21. Guyatt GH, Norris SL, Schulman S, et al. Methodology for the development of antithrombotic therapy and prevention of thrombosis guidelines: Antithrombotic Therapy and Prevention of Thrombosis, 9th ed: American College of Chest Physicians Evidence-Based Clinical Practice Guidelines. Chest 2012;141:53S–70S</bok>

22. Halani SH, Baum GR, Riley JP, et al. Esophageal perforation after anterior cervical spine surgery: a systematic review of the literature. J Neurosurg Spine 2016;25(3):285–291

23. Joaquim AF, Murar J, Savage JW, Patel AA. Dysphagia after anterior cervical spine surgery: a systematic review of potential preventative measures. Spine J 2014;14(9):2246–2260

24. Jung HJ, Park JB, Kong CG, Kim YY, Park J, Kim JB. Postoperative urinary retention following anterior cervical spine surgery for degenerative cervical disc diseases. Clin Orthop Surg 2013;5(2):134–137

25. Kaloostian PE, Kim JE, Bydon A, et al. Intracranial hemorrhage after spine surgery. J Neurosurg Spine 2013;19(3):370–380

26. Kazaure HS, Martin M, Yoon JK, Wren SM. Long-term results of a postoperative pneumonia prevention program for the inpatient surgical ward. JAMA Surg 2014;149(9):914–918

27. Konstantinides SV, Torbicki A, Agnelli G, et al; Task Force for the Diagnosis and Management of Acute Pulmonary Embolism of the European Society of Cardiology (ESC). 2014 ESC guidelines on the diagnosis and management of acute pulmonary embolism. Eur Heart J 2014;35(43):3033–3069, 3069a–3069k

28. Kyrle PA, Eichinger S. Deep vein thrombosis. Lancet 2005;365(9465):1163–1174

29. Lee TH, Lee JS, Hong SJ, et al. Risk factors for postoperative ileus following orthopedic surgery: the role of chronic constipation. J Neurogastroenterol Motil 2015;21(1):121–125

30. Nanda A, Sharma M, Sonig A, Ambekar S, Bollam P. Surgical complications of anterior cervical diskectomy and fusion for cervical degenerative disk disease: a single surgeon's experience of 1,576 patients. World Neurosurg 2014;82(6):1380–1387

31. Nandyala SV, Marquez-Lara A, Park DK, et al. Incidence, risk factors, and outcomes of postoperative airway management after cervical spine surgery. Spine 2014;39(9):E557–E563

32. Ohya J, Chikuda H, Oichi T, et al. Perioperative stroke in patients undergoing elective spinal surgery: a retrospective analysis using the Japanese diagnosis procedure combination database. BMC Musculoskelet Disord 2015;16:276

33. Palumbo MA, Aidlen JP, Daniels AH, Bianco A, Caiati JM. Airway compromise due to laryngopharyngeal edema after anterior cervical spine surgery. J Clin Anesth 2013;25(1):66–72

34. Powers WJ, Derdeyn CP, Biller J, et al; American Heart Association Stroke Council. 2015 American Heart Association/American Stroke Association Focused Update of the 2013 Guidelines for the Early Management of Patients With Acute Ischemic Stroke Regarding Endovascular Treatment: A Guideline for Healthcare Professionals From the American Heart Association/American Stroke Association. Stroke 2015;46(10):3020–3035

35. Qaseem A, Snow V, Barry P, et al; Joint American Academy of Family Physicians/American College of Physicians Panel on Deep Venous Thrombosis/Pulmonary

Embolism. Current diagnosis of venous thromboembolism in primary care: a clinical practice guideline from the American Academy of Family Physicians and the American College of Physicians. Ann Fam Med 2007;5(1):57–62

36. Roberts GW, Bekker TB, Carlsen HH, Moffatt CH, Slattery PJ, McClure AF. Postoperative nausea and vomiting are strongly influenced by postoperative opioid use in a dose-related manner. Anesth Analg 2005;101(5):1343–1348

37. Roh GU, Yang SY, Shim JK, Kwak YL. Efficacy of palonosetron versus ramosetron on preventing opioid-based analgesia-related nausea and vomiting after lumbar spinal surgery: a prospective, randomized, and double-blind trial. Spine 2014;39(9):E543–E549

38. Sagi HC, Beutler W, Carroll E, Connolly PJ. Airway complications associated with surgery on the anterior cervical spine. Spine 2002;27(9):949–953

39. Sanchez TR, Holz GS, Corwin MT, Wood RJ, Wootton-Gorges SL. Follow-up barium study after a negative water-soluble contrast examination for suspected esophageal leak: is it necessary? Emerg Radiol 2015;22(5):539–542

40. Schoenfeld AJ, Herzog JP, Dunn JC, Bader JO, Belmont PJ Jr. Patient-based and surgical characteristics associated with the acute development of deep venous thrombosis and pulmonary embolism after spine surgery. Spine 2013;38(21):1892–1898

41. Schoenfeld AJ, Ochoa LM, Bader JO, Belmont PJ Jr. Risk factors for immediate postoperative complications and mortality following spine surgery: a study of 3475 patients from the National Surgical Quality Improvement Program. J Bone Joint Surg Am 2011;93(17):1577–1582

42. Shah KN, Waryasz G, DePasse JM, Daniels AH. Prevention of paralytic ileus utilizing alvimopan following spine surgery. Orthop Rev (Pavia) 2015;7(3):6087

43. Smith JS, Saulle D, Chen CJ, et al. Rates and causes of mortality associated with spine surgery based on 108,419 procedures: a review of the Scoliosis Research Society Morbidity and Mortality Database. Spine 2012;37(23):1975–1982

44. Swann MC, Hoes KS, Aoun SG, McDonagh DL. Postoperative complications of spine surgery. Best Pract Res Clin Anaesthesiol 2016;30(1):103–120

45. Wang TY, Martin JR, Loriaux DB, et al. Risk assessment and characterization of 30-day perioperative myocardial infarction following spine surgery: a retrospective analysis of 1346 consecutive adult patients. Spine 2016;41(5):438–444

46. Willson MC, Ross JS. Postoperative spine complications. Neuroimaging Clin N Am 2014;24(2):305–326 .

# Index